No More Diets

(A Guide To Healthy Eating)

First Published in Australia by Anne Rogers

Copyright © 2005 by Anne Rogers.

Published by Lulu .com 2008

No More Diets (A Guide To Healthy Eating)

ISBN 978-1-4092-0468-8

Contact the author: jadzia1994@lizzy.com.au

Authors Website: www.annerogersbooks.com

www.lulu.com/annerogers

No More Diets (A Guide To Healthy Eating). If you could improve any aspect of your health today, what would you choose? Would you want to be at your ideal weight? Feel and look younger. Avoid premature aging? Reduce or eliminate some diseases or illness? Not feel tired all the time, increase your energy. Anne Rogers is a retired nurse (Bachelor of Arts Registered Nurse Flinders University SA) and qualified nutritionist (Diploma of Nutrition and Aesthetics SA) . She spent 10 years researching this book. She was very overweight, 18 stone while nursing and felt tired and unhealthy most of the time, and she was desperate to lose weight. Anne tried lots of diets, which failed. She decided to research and write this book after qualifying as a nutritionist; she lost weight by putting the advice in her book in to practice. Anne now weighs 10.5 stone and has more energy and feels healthier. She does not diet and eats as much as she wants and enjoys her food and her new found health. All the people who have read this book have benefited from following the advice therein and have improved their health and lost weight.

Eleven Reasons Why You Need This Book

1. With this book you will learn how to eat more healthily.
2. Learn how to live a longer healthier life.
3. Learn about the alkaline-acid balance and why it is important to your health. Which foods keep the balance correct.
4. The benefits of eating raw vegetables.
5. The danger of eating white refined food and salt and other highly processed food.
6. All about the different kinds of foods and what they can do for you.
7. Vitamins and minerals and other micro nutrients, and why they are essential for good health. And why deficiencies lead to ill health and disease.
8. Learn how to lose those kilos without going on a restrictive diet that is impossible to keep to. And why restrictive dieting can ruin your health, and end up making you fatter than ever.
9. How to make the changes in your diet and lifestyle simply and easily without tears and tantrums.
10. Why what you drink is important to your health.
11. Learn about the Glycemic index and how it can help you control your calorie intake without having to count calories. Which foods are high, medium and low on the Glycemic index.

Contents

INTRODUCTION

Five hundred years before the birth of Christ, Hippocrates the father of the natural healing sciences said 'Food will be thy medicine and medicine thy food' How right he was, there are many forms of illness which can only be successfully cured or managed by an appropriate and adequate diet. Malnutrition is far more common than you think. It doesn't just apply to those who don't have enough to eat. It can also apply to those people who live for the best part of the week on 'fast food' and 'junk food'. A person can be fat and overfed but still be mal-nourished simply from eating the wrong kind of food. The food you eat can make or break you. You can literally dig your own grave with your knife and fork. How many of us sit in front of the TV all evening drinking coffee or beer, crunching away on candy bars, tucking into hot dogs, greasy half cremated hamburgers, fried chicken and chips, cookies, cakes, doughnuts, salted peanuts, chocolates. Then at proper mealtimes load their already groaning stomach with yet more over rich food. Then to top it all off finish with a stodgy or over sugary dessert, then wash it all down with even more coffee or beer. Does this sound a little like you?

Is it any wonder people suffer the health depleting affects of such dietary insanity, or die at an early age from heart and weight related problems? Western civilized man is committing voluntary suicide on a huge scale. We are slowly but surely eating our way to extinction. However, does this have to be the case? The answer is no, of course not, surely we can be the masters of our own destiny. We don't have to continue eating ourselves to death even if our neighbors and work mates choose to. With a little effort and understanding we can live a long and healthy life simply by eating the right sort of food in adequate amounts. So from today, yes I mean right now, make the next meal you eat a healthy one. From now on take charge of your life.

CHAPTER ONE:
WHAT CAUSES WEIGHT GAIN AND DISEASE ?

THE WESTERN DIET

If we consume a traditional Western diet (and most of us do) we can expect to die in the prime of our life (50s to 70s) of some kind of degenerative disease. We call it 'dying of old age'. Practically everyone dies of old age and it is accepted as being normal. However, it is far from normal. These degenerative diseases and weight problems are the result of bad eating habits and could possibly be avoided if the diet is improved.

CHANGING A LIFETIME HABIT

The main problem to be overcome in improving the diet is kicking our addiction to the highly flavored processed foods we are so accustomed to. Because of the tempting flavors we are encouraged to eat far more than we need. The food pollutes our body with cholesterol, protein wastes and toxic by-products like salt, fat, chemical dyes and preservatives. This condition of the body which is more or less permanent on the Western diet is known as 'Lipotoxeamia' and leads to the formation of excess fat deposits and disease.

PROBLEMS START EARLY

The problem starts when we are children with weight gain, diabetes, headaches and migraine. By the time we are in the so called prime of our life (30s) we suffer from poor eyesight, arthritis, high blood pressure, obesity, circulatory problems and the beginning of heart disease. In middle age (45s) we have angina, blocked arteries, heart attack, stomach ulcers, glaucoma, diabetes, cancer and many other problems too numerous to mention. If we are lucky enough to live past our seventies we can look forward to senility, strokes and kidney failure to name but a few of the ailments of so called old age. If we don't die from all this we are most likely incapacitated by crippling arthritis or osteoporosis and must live out the rest of our miserable life in a nursing home. Many people exist in a vegetative state unable to communicate or do for themselves, with no awareness of anything around them. It is a sad fact that the medical profession has no real answers to many of the problems or diseases mentioned. It's a pretty grim picture isn't it! How many people do you know who are suffering from the effects of so called old age creeping on? Would it not be better and worth living for if we could remain active and keep all our senses? I find it quite sad to hear the responses of friends when I say to them I want to live to be 150.

Repeatedly they say 'Oh I don't, I don't want to live to that sort of age because by then I'll just be a helpless thing in a nursing home.'

Then I reply 'But what if you still had all your senses and mobility, wouldn't it be great to live such a wonderfully long life?"

Their answer is 'But I wouldn't have all my senses."

I realised then that the majority of people don't believe they will live much longer than 70 or 80 and many do not expect or wish to live that long because they believe they will be a vegetable even before they reach 70. It would seem that people have been brainwashed into thinking they cannot possibly live a long and active life because they have no control over the effects of the aging process. This is where they are wrong!

A SIMPLE SOLUTION

It may seem like too simple a solution, to say that a lot of diseases and weight problems could be avoided if the diet was improved. Happily more and more people in the health professions are turning to good nutrition to treat their patients. They are beginning to realize that diet can cure, when drugs have failed.

The body is a wonderful self healing thing, and given the chance – e.g.: freedom from toxins and optimum nutrition - will always remain healthy for that is its natural state. It is our misuse and abuse that renders it unhealthy. If more people gave their bodies as much care and attention that some people lavish on their cars we would all be a lot healthier. Let's face it you only have one body, if it breaks down you can't trade it in for a new one like you can with a car.

TEN TIPS FOR A LONGER LIFE

1. Eat smaller portions of food more often, rather than large infrequent meals. E.g.: Breakfast; snack; lunch; snack; dinner, supper.
2. Eat fruit and vegetables as fresh as possible eat raw when possible.
3. Include adequate roughage in your diet (Bran, celery, greens.)
4. Cut out organic salt (common table salt.) It gives you hardening of the arteries.
5. Eat foods rich in vitamins and minerals.
6. Eat fresh yogurt and pro-biotics (Yakult or Bios) daily.
7. Eat garlic or odorless garlic tablets or onions, to guard against colds and flu, but only if they don't cause digestive upsets
8. Avoid over eating, only eat as much as you need.
9. Eat foods containing complete proteins; but in moderation (eggs, milk, meat, fish.) unless you are a vegetarian, then eat vegetable proteins (seeds, cereals, grains, nuts, peas, legumes, baked beans and corn).
10. Balance carbohydrates with proteins at meal times.

'Life is not merely to be alive, but to be well'. (Martial.)

CHAPTER TWO:
THE DIGESTIVE SYSTEM

When you smell or think of food your mouth waters and this is the start of the digestive process. An adult will make up to 2 litres of saliva a day. Saliva consists of water, mucus and an enzyme called amylase, which breaks down starch into dextrin's. When food is swallowed it passes into the oesophagus which is about 25cm long, the food is kept moving by muscular action called peristalsis. At the end of the oesophagus is a J shaped bag called the stomach. It is sealed at both ends by muscular sphincters, the top one is called the cardiac and the bottom one is the pyloric. They prevent food from entering or leaving until the stomach is ready. The inside of the stomach is lubricated by a protective mucus, which prevents gastric juices from digesting the stomach itself. Gastric juice is made up of water, hydrochloric acid, enzymes, mucus and mineral salts. About every 20 seconds the stomach churns the food by muscular action and turns it into chyme, a creamy looking fluid. The chyme is then passed into the small intestine for absorption. The small intestine is the longest part of your digestive tract, being up to 6 meters.

The small intestine is comprised of 3 sections, the duodenum, jejunum and the ileum. Enzymes secreted by the small intestine break down the chyme so that it can be absorbed, amylase for starch, protease for protein and lipase for fat. The pancreas also makes these enzymes to help digestion and it also makes insulin. After all the nutrients have been taken out, what remains of the food enters the large intestine by the ileocecal sphincter. The large intestine plays no part in digestion it merely absorbs most of the remaining water from the food waste before it passes out of the body via the rectum and anus.

The digestive process demands large amounts of energy and some foods are harder to digest than others, they spend a long time in the stomach and require lots of energy to digest. Proteins are the hardest to digest; they require an extremely acid environment at a pH of 4.5 down to 2.0 they will stay in the stomach for many hours before they go on into the intestines. Pepsin which digests protein can only work at below pH 4.5.

Starchy foods like potato's, rice, pasta, bread and anything made with flour are easier to digest and they will only stay in the stomach for about three hours before passing into the intestines. When these foods enter the mouth they are mixed with the enzyme amylase in the saliva, this starts to digest the food straight away. When these foods enter the stomach the pH is 7.0 (neutral) and they can continue to be digested until the pH level drops to 4.5. Below this amylase can no longer work.

The non starchy vegetables are very easy to digest as well; they only stay in the stomach for about three hours. They require the same ph levels as starchy food.

The easiest food of all to digest is fruit; it is almost pre-digested and takes only 20-30 minutes in the stomach before moving on into the intestines.

'Happiness lies, first of all, in health'. (W.G. Curtis.)

CHAPTER THREE:
THE ALKALINE-ACID BALANCE

Research groups in Sweden and America have made an interesting discovery. They have found that when a person eats over 60% of the alkaline foods they get an emotional lift, they feel more alert and have more energy. Any obsessive eating habits cease and they find it easier to stop smoking.

Our blood pH is normally between 7.35 and 7.45 (slightly alkaline) which is a pretty narrow margin for error. The body is amazingly adaptable but if you constantly strain it to the limit by eating the wrong kind of food, ill health and weight gain can be the result.

The ideal diet would be to eat 60% to 80% alkaline foods. These are vegetables and fruit, millet and buckwheat. The other 40% to 20% would be the acid foods, these are animal proteins: meat, fish, eggs and dairy products, plant proteins: nuts and all starchy food, tea, coffee and alcohol.

It would seem to make sense that to stay healthy and slim we need to do two things.

1.   Correctly combine our foods so as to put less strain on the digestive system.

2. Eat more alkaline foods and less acid foods.

Some of the symptoms of over toxicity are:

☐   Furry tongue

☐   Bad breath

☐   Constant hunger

☐   Fatigue

☐   Poor skin

☐   Mood changes

☐   Irritability

☐   Depression

☐   Constant headaches and migraines

☐   Obsessive eating and/or drinking habits

ALKALINE FOODS

Asparagus

Beetroot

Broccoli

Brussels Sprouts

Cabbage

Capsicum

Carrots

Cauliflower

Celery

Cucumber

Eggplant

Lettuce

Leek

Mushrooms

Onion

Buckwheat

Silverbeat

Spinach

Tomato

Zucchini

Sprouts

ACID FOODS

Red and white meat

Dairy products

Eggs

Meat by-products

Fish

Seeds

Beans

Peas

Nuts

Soy

Coconut

Rice

Pasta

Flour

Bread

Cereals

Plums

ALKALINE FRUIT

Apples

Apricots

Avacado

Bananna

Cherries

Figs

Grapefruit

Grapes

Kiwifruit

Lemons

Manderins

Mangoes

Rockmelon

Necterines

Oranges

Passionfruit

Peaches

Pears

Pineapple

Rockmelon

Rhubarb

Strawberries

Limes

Watermelon

Paw paw

Honeydew Melon

THE BENEFITS OF EATING RAW VEGETABLES

By eating raw vegetables you will be providing your body with the very best possible nourishment. Raw vegetables if eaten when they are fresh, contain enzymes which make them very easy to digest and some enzymes will be available to help with the bodies internal enzyme needs. They are also full of vitamins and minerals. Because raw vegetables are easy to digest they put less strain on the digestive system, passing through the stomach in only two hours. Cooking or heating vegetables destroys the enzymes and also some of the vitamins. It also destroys most of the taste. Raw vegetables all have their unique flavours which can be quite strong and delicious. You will gain the most benefit from your vegetables if you eat as many raw vegetables as possible. If you have trouble chewing raw vegetables chop them finely then put them into a blender or food processer, do each vegetable seperately so that the individual flavours are retained.

SPROUTED SEEDS, GRAINS AND LEGUMES

Sprouted seeds, grains and legumes are some of the most nutritionaly valuable foods there are, they are also some of the easiest foods to digest. Sprouted seeds, grains and legumes supply all the necessary elements of nutrition; all the essential amino acids (protein), natural sugars (carbohydrates) and the essential fatty acids. They are also full of enzymes and vitamins in a highly concentrated form.

Seeds, grains and legumes in the unsprouted form are acid forming and contain enzyme inhibitors which suspend the life cycle of the seed until conditions are favourable for growth. This inhibitor prevents the enzymes and vitamins from being digested and also makes the seed very hard to digest at all. Cooking destroys the inhibitor and makes the seed easier to digest, but it also destroys the enzymes and some of the vitamins, so they are less nutritious.

'He who has good health is young'. (H.G. Bohn.)

CHAPTER FOUR:
REFINED FOOD GOOD OR BAD?

REFINED WHITE SUGAR

Not only is it worthless as an item of nourishment, it is also very bad for the health consumed in great quantities. In deserts, beverages, sweets, ice-cream and cakes. However the greatest thing to condemn refined white sugar is its high solubility in the body, it is a high GI food, it rushes in with little time to be digested, stimulating excess secretions of insulin by the pancreas causing it to go into overdrive to deal with the imbalance that has been created. Have you ever experienced a kind of sick yucky feeling after eating something that was very sweet. If you have you are experiencing Hyperglycaemia a condition that is caused through too much sugar in your blood stream. It passes off after a while when your poor overworked pancreas has pumped out enough Insulin to deal with the overload. After a while the blood sugar drops but because of the excess of insulin that was needed your blood sugar levels can drop too low and you may then experience Hypoglycaemia, with weakness, shaking and a nasty sick feeling once again.

If you must use sugar try raw brown sugar or honey which contains enzymes that are good for the digestion.

REFINED WHITE FLOUR

Also worthless as a food item. It has had all its natural goodness refined out of it, leaving only great stuff for making glue. You will be much better off eating whole grain flour.

SALT

Inorganic sodium chloride or common table salt is a killer! Why? Because it is indigestible, the body simply doesn't have the means to deal with large amounts of inorganic substances. So what happens to all that salt so liberally sprinkled over the veggie's before cooking, the chips, the salad? Well it must either be eliminated or stored in water soluble form. This overloads the kidneys and waterlogs the body tissues. We've all heard of water retention, practically everyone suffers from it to some degree or other. What's the first thing you lose when you go on a diet? Yes, you guessed it. Water!

Salt also contributes to high blood pressure and that can lead to atherosclerosis (blocked blood vessels) and hardening of the arteries (which become narrower and stiffer) which strain the heart. Salt also paralyses the 260 taste buds in the mouth ruining your sense of taste. That's why people often say they don't like vegetables, they have no taste. These people are usually users of salt, no wonder they can't taste their veggie's, their taste buds are asleep! It takes up to three months for your taste buds to wake up after you stop using salt, so be patient.

Salt is also addictive and can cause nervous tension, insomnia and migraine. But don't get me wrong, our bodies need salt, but we get all the salt we need from fresh fruit and vegetables in the form of organic sodium.

'The smaller your waistline, the longer your lifeline'. (Anon.)

CHAPTER FIVE:
DIFFERENT TYPES OF FOOD

PROTEINS – THE BODIES MAINTENANCE TEAM

Protein is the basic raw material of all living things, everything around you that is alive, the plants and animals and even ourselves are constructed from protein. Our bodies are made of many kinds of tissues and the tissues are formed out of different types of cells. They form your hair, skin, teeth, bones, nails, heart, kidneys, liver, brain, eyes, nerves and muscles and all the other parts of your body. Every last ounce of you is made of protein. So you can see that if your body should lack protein it is going to have a hard time keeping things running smoothly. As each little protein cell wears out and dies it must be replaced by a new one. If the cells aren't replaced then things start to go wrong. For instance the immune system would be affected, this vital system is made up of anti-bodies which are complex molecules constructed from amino acids (protein) to deal with invading organisms. A lack of protein could mean a lack of anti-bodies leading to you catching colds, flu and gastric flu and all the other ailments going the rounds. Or you could catch something far worse. As for the other affects of insufficient protein, nails become brittle, hair and skin become dry, muscles become weak and you would become anaemic. A lack of protein could lead to over eating and over weight if the diet is too low in protein and too high in carbohydrates.

Higher protein meals needn't be expensive if you pick the cheaper cuts of meat and cook them slowly to tenderise them, a kilo of minced beef can go a long way. An omelette is a protein packed cheap meal, a chicken costs no more than a fancy cake and will be much healthier for you. So what are these protein foods? Well top of the list comes meat, the usual muscle meat and organ meat such as heart and brains (liver and kidneys are not recommended they contain too many toxins). Chicken and fish, then milk and eggs, butter, cheese and yoghurt are all good protein foods. Then there are things like seeds, cereals, grains, nuts, peas, beans, baked beans, corn, sunflower seeds and millet all eaten in their natural state (that is unprocessed) are high in protein. However vegetable protein is not as effective as animal protein. Add some carbohydrates and you have a balanced diet and a healthy body able to fight disease and repair damage, keep the skin and hair in good condition and muscles strong with plenty of energy.

CARBOHYDRATES – FUEL FOR THE FURNACE

What did you have for your evening meal yesterday? Some lovely stodgy dumplings with steak and kidney, or was it a plate full of delicious mashed potato with lashings of butter to fill up the gaps. What about desert? A generous helping of chocolate pudding and lovely thick custard or maybe it was ice-cream and jelly. Watch out !!!!!!!!!!!!!! Although we need carbohydrates in our diet too much of the wrong sort and they could turn out to be killers.

What exactly are carbohydrates? To put it simply they are starches and sugars. If you are the average person who up until now has never really worried about what you eat, or stopped to consider the affects your diet has on your health, then you probably eat up to 75% more carbohydrates than are good for you.

The very worst sort of carbohydrates are the things like stodgy dumplings made with refined white flour, chocolate pudding, custard (yellow glue) and ice-cream and jelly, (refined white sugar and coloured water that sets solid) fruit pies, rice pudding and cakes.

So what sort of carbohydrates are good for you? That's easy, the sort found in fresh vegetables, fruit, milk, pasta, whole grains and cereals. They also contain protein, vitamins and minerals. Things which are completely missing from the refined starches and sugars.

But you might be thinking potatoes have just been condemned and that's true, in larges amounts, but in moderation the humble potato can take it's place along with the other vegetables. Carbohydrates provide energy but in order to stay slim and healthily active we need protein as well. Filling up with heavy starchy food thinking it will give more energy is a misconception. Heavy starchy meals won't make you feel lively and alert, on the conterary it will do quite the reverse. So what happens to all these excess carbohydrates you've just consumed? They won't be burned up as energy, all you want to do right now is flop in the armchair and sleep it off. They'll be stored as fat, and if you continue your daily diet of stodge you'll continue to store more and more fat. Once it's there it's very hard to dislodge.

FATS FOR ENERGY

A certain amount of fat is needed in the healthy diet. Fat provides the body with energy, twice as much in fact as an equal amount of carbohydrates. Plant oils such as palm, olive, sunflower and safflower oils contain vitamin E. All fats contain vitamins, they also help to insulate the body, fat protects vital organs. The saturated fats are found in butter, milk, cheese and fat on meat; they are the culprits they are converted into cholesterol and should be used sparingly as a high cholesterol level in the body can lead to blocked arteries and heart attack. The best fats are the mon-un-saturated fats from seeds, grains and olive oil. There is a lot of controversy over poly un-saturated fats these days. One eye specialist uses only olive oil, he says poly un-saturated oils such as canola and rape seed contain an acid which causes de-genarative eye disease (Macular Degeneration). Poly un-saturated oil is also found in safflower, peanut and soy beans. To cut down the fat content in milk or soy milk use fat reduced. To cut down the fat in cheese, butter or margarine use the fat reduced varieties. A handy tip, if you don't like the taste of fat reduced milk or soy milk mix a litre of full fat with a litre of fat reduced, it will taste better and you will have cut your fat intake by a little less than half.

CHAPTER SIX:
VITAMINS – ESSENTIAL FOR HEALTH

Vitamins

What are vitamins? Vitamins are an organic food substance found only in living things such as plants and animals. Vitamins are vital for life, if we had to go without certain vitamins we would become very sick or die. A well known vitamin deficiency is scurvy (lack of vitamin C) another is rickets (lack of vitamin D). If the body is deprived of all the vitamins we would most certainly die.

There are two types of vitamins the water soluble vitamins B, C, P and the fat soluble vitamins A, D, E, F, and K.

The fat soluble vitamins.

Vitamin A

Retinal this vitamin is found in parsley, carrots and pumpkin. Also in cod liver oil, butter fat, cream, full milk, cheese, eggs and liver. It protects the mucus membranes of the mouth, nose and throat, lungs, digestive tract and kidneys against infection. Helps to form strong bones and teeth and maintains good vision. A word of warning don't rush out and buy some vitamin A tablets, too much will make you ill. Because it is fat soluble the body stores it in the liver, an overdose can lead to a toxic build up and swelling of the liver. If you eat the right kind of food you should get all the vitamin A your body needs. It doesn't require vitamin A every day unlike the water soluble vitamins B or C which aren't stored and get flushed out daily.

Vitamin D

This vitamin is often called the 'sunshine' vitamin but we don't actually get vitamin D from the sun. What happens is, exposure to ultra-violet rays stimulate the body to manufacture vitamin D. We also get it from cod liver oil, liver, milk, butter and cheese. Vitamin D is essential for strong teeth and bones in growing children; a lack of it causes rickets (soft weak bones). It works together with calcium and helps the blood to clot in cases of cuts and wounds. It also helps the relaxation of the nerves.

Vitamin E

D-alpha-tocopherol is found in cold pressed vegetable oils, seed oil, nut and grain oil. It is good for increasing muscular tone as it improves cellular respiration in the muscle tissues. Vitamin E also helps the healing of scar tissue, can ward off miscarriages by stabilizing the hormones. Deficiencies can lead to thrombosis, sterility, muscular dystrophy and hemorrhoids.

Vitamin F

This is a fat soluble un-saturated fatty acid and is found in soy beans, corn, safflower and seed oils. It helps to break up deposits of cholesterol, helps blood clotting and keeps the skin and mucus membranes lubricated. Deficiencies cause dry skin, dry hair and nails, allergies, dermatitis and acne.

Vitamins K1 and K2

These vitamins can be found in yogurt, full milk, egg yolk, fish, liver, oils, green leafy vegetables and meat. Vitamins K1 and K2 are essential for blood clotting. However taking extra doses by way of a supplement is not advised as sufficient amounts are obtained in the normal diet.

The water soluble Vitamins

Vitamin C

Ascorbic Acid is essential for the formation of healthy connective tissue such as ligaments and bones. It helps the healing of wounds and prevents hemorrhaging and gingivitis (gum disease). Vitamin C is found in citrus fruits, vegetables, rosehips, green and red capsicums. The body doesn't store Vitamin C so a daily intake is needed especially in cases of illness such as colds, flu and throat infections. Deficiencies can cause scurvy, bruising, bleeding gums, nose bleed, slow healing wounds, weak capillaries and painful swollen joints. Vitamin C must be taken with vitamins P (bioflavonoids) otherwise the body doesn't absorb vitamin C properly.

Vitamins P

These vitamins are commonly known as bioflavonoids, there are two, Rutin which comes from buckwheat and Hesperidin which comes from citrus. Vitamin C and P work together controlling the permeability of the tissues. Deficiencies lead to weak capillaries, hemorrhaging and bruising. Vitamin P should be taken in conjunction with Vitamin C for proper absorption of C.

Vitamins B

B1 (Thiamin), B2 (Riboflavin), Folic Acid, Para Aminobenzoic Acid, B3 (Niacin), B5 (Pantothenic Acid), B6 (Paradoxin Hydrochloride), B12 (Cyanocobalamin). The B vitamins are important for the production of energy they are vital for the formation of enzymes in the digestive tract. Protein and B vitamins combine to produce enzymes. B vitamins do not exist naturally as individuals; each one must rely on the others for its action. Therefore it is no good to just take one of the B vitamins on its own thinking it will do you good, the whole complex must be taken to reap the benefits from them. B vitamins can be found in brewers yeast powder, liver, dairy products and green leafy vegetables. B1 is needed for healthy nerves and improving and stabilizing the digestion. B2 for healthy skin and production of enzymes for digestion. B3 for good circulation and it is an anti-inflammatory. Folic Acid for healthy cell growth and repair, especially for pregnant women. Para Aminobenzoic Acid for healthy skin and hair and protects the skin from ultra-violet rays. B5 an anti-stress vitamin and protects the body from radiation. B6 for proper relaxation and sleep, helps to alleviate premenstrual tension. B12 for nourishment of the nervous system and essential for the brain cells. B vitamins can prevent diabetic nerve damage. Deficiencies in B vitamins can lead to mental fatigue, irritability, herpes, sensitive eyes, worms, impaired mental development in children, exhaustion, inflamed skin and joints, morning sickness, migraine, pernicious aneamia and disturbance of the nervous system. B complex vitamins should be taken daily as these vitamins are not stored by the body.

SOURCES OF VITAMINS

A – Parsley, carrots, pumpkin, cod liver oil, butter fat, cream, full milk, cheese, eggs and liver.

Bs – Brewers yeast powder, liver, dairy products, green leafy vegetables.

C – Citrus fruit, vegetables, rosehips, green and red capsicums.

D – Cod liver oil, liver, milk, butter, and cheese.

E – Cold pressed vegetable oils, seed oil, nut and grain oil.

F – Soya, corn, safflower oil, seed oil.

Ks – Yogurt, full milk, egg yolk, fish, liver, vegetable oils, green leafy vegetables and meat.

Ps – Buckwheat, citrus fruit, grapes, blackcurrants, plums and blackberries.

CHAPTER: SEVEN
MINERALS AND ENZYMES

MINERALS

Minerals are inorganic substances that are found in all living things such as animals and plants. They work in harmony with other essential life giving nutrients. A deficiency of one mineral may disrupt the entire chain of life, rendering other nutrients useless or inefficient. There are close to 30 known minerals, all of which influence your health and personality. Of these 14 dominate the health picture. Each of these minerals need the other minerals, for together they influence vitamins, proteins, amino acids, enzymes, carbohydrates, fats, and sugars. Minerals can either build or destroy an entire person, depending upon their supply or deficiency. Some minerals exert a specific action on a specific body function. Magnesium is natures tranquilizer; Sulphur acts as an overall beauty treatment. All minerals are required to build and maintain mental and physical vigor.

Calcium

This mineral must have vitamins A, C and D and phosphorus in order to function, these other nutrients must have Calcium to do their work properly. About 99% of your Calcium is found in your bones and teeth. Calcium works to normalize the contraction and relaxation of the heart muscles. If your blood calcium level drops too low you become nervous and irritated. An adequate supply of Calcium is required for the proper functioning of your brain, if there is not enough your memory will be impaired and problem solving will be difficult. Other deficiencies include osteoporosis (brittle bones), rickets (weak bones). Sources of Calcium are dairy products, green vegetables and bone meal.

Phosphorus

You will find this mineral in all of your body cells. About 66% of body Phosphorus is in the bones in a form known as Calcium Phosphate, 33% is in soft tissue as organic and inorganic Phosphate. This mineral converts oxidative energy to cell work. Phosphorus sparks internal energy. It works to neutralize excess blood acidity, it also helps create lecithin and cerebrin, ingredients needed for mental power, and it metabolizes fats and starches. A deficiency may cause appetite and weight loss, nervous disorder, mental sluggishness and general fatigue. In extreme cases, irregular breathing and a pale wan appearance. Avoid white refined sugar; the delicate calcium-phosphorus balance is interfered with in the presence of white sugar. Sources of this mineral are bone meal and supplements.

Iron

Billions of your body cells and tissues need Iron for life giving oxygen. Without Iron, about 300 litres of blood, rather than the 8 or so litres would be necessary to handle the bodies oxygen needs. Iron is found in the red blood cells, it influences proteins and must have Calcium and the other nutrients in order to function properly. Deficiencies can cause sore cracked lips, poor memory and an inability to think clearly. Anaemia and a lack of energy along with a 'washed out' feeling. Sources of Iron include egg yolks, green leafy vegetables, molasses, plums, cherries, sun dried raisins, red meat and liver.

Iodine

This mineral stimulates the thyroid gland to secrete the hormone thyroxin that regulates energy and metabolism. Deficiencies can cause goiter, obesity, sluggish metabolism and lowered mentality, rapid pulse, heart palpitation, tremor, nervousness, restlessness and irritability. Iodine is needed to utilize fat and influence other nutrients. It is found in foods such as fish, kelp, dehydrated sea weed, dulse and onions.

Sodium

This mineral works with Potassium to help maintain the favorable acid-base factor in your body. It also helps maintain a normal water level balance between cells and fluids. A deficiency can cause stomach and intestinal gas and poor digestion of carbohydrates, weight loss and muscle shrinkage. Sodium favors the formation and free flow of saliva, gastric juices and enzymes. It is found in sea foods, poultry, beet, carrots, chard and dandelion greens.

Potassium

Another balancing mineral, it works with sodium to normalize the heart beat and feed the muscles. It joins with Phosphorus to send oxygen to the brain. Sodium and Potassium have to be balanced. Potassium is found mostly inside the cells, a small amount is outside them. It stimulates the kidneys to dispose of body wastes. A deficiency can lead to constipation, nervous disorder, insomnia, slow irregular heart beat and muscle damage, enlarged kidneys and brittle bones. Deficiency of potassium and sodium can occur in people taking fluid tablets. Sources include citrus fruits, watercress, mint leaves, green capsicums, chicory, blackstrap molasses and figs.

Magnesium

This mineral is closely related to both Calcium and Phosphorus in its locations and its functions in the body. About 70% of the Magnesium in the body is in the bones; the rest is in the soft tissues and blood. Magnesium acts as a starter for some chemical reactions within the body. It plays an important role as a co-enzyme in the building of protein. Magnesium, by cooling the muscular structure during hot weather acts as a natural cooling system. Deficiencies can cause an exaggerated sensitivity to noise, dilation of blood vessels, rapid heart beat and nervousness. Sources are beet greens, cucumber, cauliflower, sunflower seeds, figs, lemons, grapefruit, corn, almonds, oil rich nuts, seeds, wild rice, apples, celery and vegetable oils. Magnesium and calcium can help to relieve muscle cramps.

Copper

Although Iron is used to make blood, Copper must also be present to convert Iron into haemoglobin. This mineral influences Tyrosine an amino acid and utilizes vitamin C. A deficiency causes anaemia, easy bone fractures, skin sores that will not heal, general weakness and impaired respiration. Copper is found in almonds, dried beans, peas, whole wheat, prunes, calf and beef liver, egg yolks, and shrimp.

Selenium

This mineral is important for maintaining cell membranes and all of the bodies cells. It is found in muscle meat, seafood and cereal. Deficiencies can cause heart disease and some cancers.

Sulphur

This mineral is natures beauty mineral; it keeps hair glossy and smooth, your skin smooth and youthful. It acts by invigorating the blood stream, causes the liver to secret bile for digestion, maintains overall body balance and has an influence on brain power. It works with B complex vitamins needed for metabolism and strong nerve health. Sources of this mineral include fish, eggs, cabbage, lean beef, dried beans and Brussels sprouts.

Silicon

It is found in hair, muscles, nails, cellular walls and connective tissues. Silicon joins with other minerals to create tooth enamel and build strong bones. Sources are buckwheat, mushrooms, carrots, tomato's, liver, whole grains and lentils.

Zinc

This mineral is a constituent of Insulin and the male reproductive fluid. It combines with Phosphorus to aid in respiration, it sparks vitamin action, and Zinc produces energy. Insulin is dependent on Zinc for proper function, an Insulin shortage causes Diabetes, Zinc helps food to be absorbed through the intestinal wall. It helps maintain healthy skin, hair and nails. A deficiency causes fatigue and poor reactions. It can be found in most shellfish, legumes and most of the foods already mentioned especially liver.

Chromium

This mineral helps to lower blood glucose levels and reduces cholesterol in people with diabetes. Chromium works as an appetite suppressant for people trying to lose weight when used with a calorie controlled diet and exercise.

Manganese

A mineral that works with the B complex vitamins to overcome lethargy and sterility. It combines with phosphatase (an enzyme) to build strong bones. It is needed for good enzymatic function so food can be digested and vital nutrients extracted for utilization. Manganese helps build resistance to disease, helps build strong nerve health, and in expectant mothers promotes milk formation. Found in most foods.

Chlorine

This mineral acts by stimulating the liver to filter waste substances from the body. Chlorine helps in keeping a youthful joint and tendon condition. A deficiency may cause hair and teeth loss, poor muscular contractions and poor digestion. Sources include kelp, dulse, sea greens, leafy green vegetables, rye flour and ripe olives.

Fluorine

Natural Fluorine helps to strengthen tooth enamel, but this is a tricky mineral. Too much can lead to unsightly tooth mottling. Small amounts are evenly distributed throughout the body tissues. Fluorine can be found in most of the foods already mentioned. It must be noted that when taken in excess, bones become weak and there is an adverse reaction upon internal organs.

ENZYMES

The word enzyme is derived from the Greek 'enzymes' meaning 'leaven' to cause change. Enzymes are catalysts, they have the power to cause an internal reaction without themselves being transformed or destroyed in the course of the process. An enzyme is an internal juice formed by living tissues and cells of the digestive tract. The body has more than 700 different types of enzymes, each one performing a separate function. A single drop of blood contains aprox 100,000 enzyme particles. Enzymes are spread throughout your entire body helping to keep you alive, a deficiency in one or more vital enzymes could lead to ill health. Without enzymes your food could not be digested to release valuable vitamins, minerals and amino acids needed to keep you alive. The Salivary glands, pancreas, stomach and intestinal walls contain digestive enzymes, there are still more enzymes in the body cells to utilize the digested nutrients passing into the system. In short enzymes perform the function of building and maintaining life and health. The body manufactures enzymes but needs to be healthy to do it. Optimally to stay healthy we need fresh air, water and food such as fruit, vegetables, eggs, milk, meat and fish in other words a balanced diet.

SOURCES OF MINERALS

Calcium – Dairy products, green leafy vegetables, oranges, figs and bone meal.

Phosphorus – Bone meal and supplements.

Iron – Egg yolk, green leafy vegetables, molasses, plums, cherries, sun dried raisins, liver and red meat.

Iodine – Fish, kelp, dehydrated sea weed, dulse and onions.

Sodium – Sea foods, poultry, beet, carrots, chard and dandelion greens.

Potassium – Citrus fruit, watercress, mint, green capsicums, chicory, blackstrap molasses, figs, bananas and dried apricots.

Magnesium – Beet greens, cucumber, cauliflower, sunflower seeds, figs lemons, grapefruit, corn, almonds, oil rich nuts, and seeds, wild rice, apples, celery and vegetable oils.

Copper – Almonds, dried beans, peas, whole wheat, prunes, liver, egg yolk and shrimp.

Sulphur – Fish, eggs, cabbage, lean beef, dried beans and Brussels sprouts.

Zinc and Manganese – Most foods and liver.

Chlorine – Kelp, dulse, sea greens, leafy green vegetables, rye flour and ripe olives.

Fluorine – Water and most foods.

'The first wealth is health'. (Emerson)

CHAPTER EIGHT:
HOW TO LOSE THE FAT

1. Eat sufficient protein.
2. Cut out fried food.
3. Cut down on carbohydrates.
4. Eat Plenty of fresh fruit and vegetables.
5. Eat low GI food.
6. Take regular exercise, at least ½ hr to 1 hr per day.

Some of the fattening Carbohydrates

Biscuits	Candy
Cake	Doughnuts
Dumplings	Éclairs
Gravy	Ice-cream
Icing	Jelly
Lasagna	Marshmallows
Pasta	Pies
Pasties	Puddings
'Quick' cereals	Refined white flour
Refined white sugar	White sauce
Yorkshire pudding	Long grain white rice
White potato	Custard
White sugar	

Some of the slimming vegetables and fruits

Asparagus	Apples
Broccoli	Apricots
Cabbage	Blackberries

Cauliflower	Blueberries
Celery	Cherries
Chinese Cabbage	Cranberries
Cucumber	Currents
Lettuce	Gooseberries
Mushrooms	Grapefruit
Artichokes	Lemons
Green Beans	Limes
Brussels Sprouts	Loganberries
Carrots	Melons
Onions	Oranges
Capsicum	Peaches
Pears	Sweet Potato
Pineapple	Rutabaga
Plums	Raspberries
Tomato	Rhubarb
Zucchini	Strawberries

Fluids vital for health

Many of us do not drink enough. A man weighing 150lbs (67.50 Kilos) is almost 75% water. Muscles are 75 – 80% water, 85% of the gray matter of the brain is water. All life processes start in water and must continue in water. Water helps cleanse and flush impurities from the body. To neglect regular water drinking between meals will leave the body wide open to many harmful conditions. Toxic wastes build up in vital organs causing damage, the tissues get clogged with debris and cellulite forms, the skin becomes congested causing spots and other blemishes. Try to make it a habit to drink at least 2 litres of pure water daily, drink more if possible. What's that I hear you cry? 'I don't like the taste of water!' Ok I'll make it a little easier on you, how about ½ water and ½ fruit juice or cordial buy the ones that are 'diet' and no added sugar, too much sugar will make you fat. Get yourself a ½ litre glass then you only have to fit 4 glasses into your day. Here's an example: one glass at breakfast time instead of coffee/tea: one glass at lunch time instead of coffee/tea: one glass at tea time instead of coffee/tea: one glass in the evening after dinner instead of coffee/tea. If you want to have coffee or tea you can drink it in between the glasses of water/fruit juice/cordial, it is recommended that you do not drink more than one glass of fruit juice per day, the rest of the day have diet cordial and water. Try to cut down on coffee it will pollute your body, no more than three ordinary size cups (250 ml). If you do that you will have consumed more than 2 litres of fluid without any difficulty. Fruit juice is good for you and there are many flavors to choose you can also make your own combinations of flavors by mixing them. Fruit juice acts as a tonic neutralizing the toxic condition of the blood and clearing body waste, they also cater for the bodies need for natural sugars, vitamins and minerals. Do not however overdo it, too much and it will make you fat or prevent you from losing the weight. Skim/low fat milk is another good drink being full of protein and other important nutrients but without the artery clogging cholesterol of full milk. The same can be said for low fat soy milk. Try to cut down on coffee no more than 2 or 3 cups a day or drink decaffeinated. Try **Nescafe Decafe** it's water filtered to remove the caffeine. Other brands use chemicals to remove the caffeine. Caffeine is addictive and depletes the bodies supply of vitamin C. Also try to cut down on tea for the same reasons, try herbal tea instead or decaffeinated.

THREE TYPES OF DIET

Lacto – Ovo – Diet (Vegetarian)
This diet includes all food except animal flesh. The foods eaten include animal by-products, eggs, milk, fruit, vegetables, nuts, grains, legumes and seeds. The diet lacks vitamin B12 which is vital for healing of wounds and for growth in pregnancy. It is recommended that a B–complex supplement should be taken.
Vega Diet

The same as the vegetarian diet but no animal by-products, strictly plant foods only.

Omnivore (Western Diet)

This diet includes all foods meat and meat by-products plus all the other vegetable foods already mentioned.

How can you tell if you are overweight?

A simple test to tell if you are overweight is to pinch up the skin behind the upper arm, between the elbow and the shoulder. If you can pinch up more than 1 inch then you are overweight.

'The best doctor in the world is doctor diet'. (Swift.)

CHAPTER NINE:
YOUR BODIES NATURAL 24 HOUR CYCLE

The human body is made up of about 75% water (blood and interstitial fluids). Water is the most important element of life; everyday we need to replenish the water we excrete in urine and sweat. Without water we would very quickly die. Because we have to replace the water we use each day the ideal diet for a human would be a diet that is 70 – 80% high water content, namely fruit and vegetables. The other 20 – 30% of our diet would be made up of the concentrated foods, those which have no water content.

Every day our body goes through a cycle, most of us are not aware of what is happening, we are so wrapped up in our daily activities. When something goes wrong you very soon become aware. For example you may become constipated and cannot use your bowels for several days, or if you get an upset stomach and have diarrhea. Your normal body cycles can become apparent if you take the time to observe what is happening on a daily basis. During the morning the body gets rid of waste products, in the day you feel hungry so you eat, at night when you are asleep the body assimilates the food you have eaten. If that normal cycle is disturbed by erratic eating and sleeping habits then your body struggles to keep the balance. If for instance you don't take proper meal breaks, or if you work shifts that are constantly changed then the normal cycles are thrown into confusion. The result is ill health and perhaps weight gain, you may not notice it at first but as the years go by it takes its toll on your general health. Most people put it down to old age creeping on, but it's not, it can be put right if you change your eating habits. One way to improve health and lose weight is to get rid of the toxins in your body. Where do these toxins come from? There are two ways that toxins are produced. Toxins are produced through the bodies natural process of metabolism. Old worn out cells die and are replaced by new ones. Every day between three hundred billion and eight hundred billion cells die. The dead cells become toxic as they break down and must be removed from the body as quickly as possible or they would poison you. There are four elimination routes, the bowels, bladder, lungs and skin. Normally this elimination process goes on without any conscious effort, but, if there is a hold up for some reason the result can mean ill health and/or weight gain. Toxins are also produced by the by-products of the food we eat. These days nearly every type of food we consume has been changed in some way from its original form before it enters our mouth. It has either been processed or refined or cooked. Hardly anything we eat is the way nature intended it to be, if we eat mostly these kinds of foods then the elimination system can't keep up, it becomes overloaded and the result is once again ill health and/or weight gain.

You can see the results of poor eating habits all around you every day. Next time you go to the supermarket to shop try counting the number of overweight people you see. Actually it would be easier to count the slim people, there are not so many of them. If you could keep your body as free of toxins as possible and the alkaline/acid balance correct you would increase your chances of staying healthy and keep slim at the same time. But how can you do it? By eating predominantly high water content food, (fruit and vegetables) and alkaline foods (see lists on pages 14-15) and drinking water, fruit and vegetable juice; you will be continuously cleansing your body of toxins and acids, never allowing the debilitating effects of toxemia and acidity to damage your body. Recent studies by scientists have shown that a diet that is predominantly fresh fruit and vegetables can lower cholesterol levels significantly in a short space of time.

EXERCISE

Any sort of program to lose weight or improve health is more effective if you incorporate some sort of exercise into it. Exercise burns glucose and this is what turns into fat if you don't use it up fairly quickly. Apart from getting you fit and helping you lose weight exercise has other benefits. It will give you a sense of well-being so that life is more enjoyable, studies have shown that exercise, fresh air and sunshine can alleviate depression; it may even prolong your life. The minimum amount of exercise for benefits is about 20 minutes 3 times a week, however for maximum benefit longer periods are recommended more often. E.g. jogging for 30 minutes – 1 hour from 4 – 7 days per week, brisk walking for 45 minutes – 1 hour from 4 – 7 days per week. You should raise your heart rate above the normal rate to get a cardiovascular effect.

- **Aerobic Exercise**

   Means 'with air', this type of exercise improves your cardiovascular ability to supply oxygen to the muscles and other parts of the body. Some of the types of aerobic exercise are walking, jogging, swimming, cycling, aerobic dance and aqua-aerobics.

- **Anaerobic Exercise**

   Means 'without air', this type of exercise increases the muscle strength and ability to cope when there is not enough oxygen. It also increases flexibility. The types of anaerobic exercise are body building, weight lifting, circuit training and free weights.

- **Flexibility Exercises**

   If you don't put your body through a full range of movement on a regular basis it will get stiffer with age. This may reduce your mobility and make you more likely to suffer damage to joints in later years. The best types of flexibility exercises are yoga, stretch and flex classes, ballet classes and any of the weight training exercises. Many people say that weight training does not do anything for your flexibility and it even makes you stiff. The author has found these statements to be false. On the contrary when I was doing only yoga I was quite stiff and found it difficult to do quite a few of the exercises. However when I took up weight training I found it improved my flexibility and strength to such a degree I was able to do yoga exercises that I had previously found virtually impossible.

'A healthy body is the guest chamber of the soul; a sick one it's prison'. (Bacon)

CHAPTER TEN:
CAN YOU EXTEND YOUR LIFE-SPAN ?

Experts on aging divide it into 2 types.

1. Primary Ageing which starts when we are young and goes on throughout life.

2. Secondary Ageing due to disease, abuse and disuse of the body.

You may not be able to effect the first type of ageing but it is possible to effect the second type of ageing. With a healthy diet and adequate exercise, diseases like cancer, diabetes and heart disease could be avoided and thus ones life might be extended.

What is normal life expectancy? In the days of the Roman Empire up to the Middle Ages a person could only expect to live for 20 or 30 years. By the mid 1800's a person could expect to reach 40 before dying. How things have changed, now a person can expect to live to around 75 years for a man and around 80 years for a woman. If cancer, heart and kidney disease could be eliminated from the picture, people could expect to add another 11 years to their life-span. That's 86 for men and 91 for women.

THE VALUE OF EATING FRUIT AND VEGETABLES

- Fat content is low.
- Dietary fibre is high.
- Salt content is low.
- Potassium content is high.
- High in vitamins and minerals.
- Beta-carotene content is high.
- Source of Folate.
- Helps prevent cancer.

- Builds up the immune system.
- Low in kilojoules.
- Helps prevent obesity.
- Helps to control diabetes.
- Most are low GI
- Lowers Cholesterol.
- Lowers blood pressure.
- Prevents bowel disorders.
- Improves elimination.

SOME EASY GUIDELINES

1. If possible eat fruit raw, don't cook it, it becomes acid. Also eat lots of raw vegetables; cooking destroys the enzymes and most of the vitamins.

2. Conserve your energy for detoxification – by eating easy to digest food during the day.

3. Don't eat meat more than once a day and then only at the evening meal. This will ensure you have plenty of time to digest it during the night. Always cut off all fat, it is high in saturated fat which causes the formation of cholesterol which clogs arteries and causes heart attacks.

4. Eat the more concentrated foods at the end of the day.

5. If you feel hungry between meals eat fruit. Or raw vegetables.

6. Eat a good variety of foods.

7. Cut down on meat consumption, it will deplete your energy levels. Meat requires a lot of energy to digest. Try eating meat or fish only three times a week. On the other days eat just vegetables. It will give your digestive tract a well earned rest. It will also help to balance your acid-alkaline levels.

8. Try to eat low fat or fat free yogurt, fat reduced cheese and margarine or butter. Drink fat reduced milk or soy milk.

9. Drink a pro-biotic like Yakult™ or Bios™ every day to keep your digestive tract healthy. Pro-biotics replace the friendly bacteria in the stomach and

small intestine that are destroyed by chlorine in drinking water and antibiotics.

10. Cut down on cheese, peanuts and eggs they are high in fat, eat in moderation.

11. If you break the rules for one meal don't panic, just make up for it in your next meal by eating properly It's what you eat most of the time that will make the difference.

12. Eat regularly don't skip meals on a regular basis.

13. Drink purified, distilled or filtered water. If you don't have a purifier get a filter bottle (they are really cheap). Tap water, spring water and tank water contain toxins and heavy metals that are bad for you.

14. Drink caffeine free beverages like herbal tea, decaffeinated tea or coffee (without sugar or use sugar substitutes), vegetable and fruit juice with no added sugar. Don't drink soft drinks or cordial (they are loaded with sugar) use diet varieties instead.

15. Drink alcohol in moderation or not at all.

16. Always drink 2 or more litres of fluid a day.

17. Cut out salt, it will cause hardening of your arteries, which leads to high blood pressure.

18. Cut out fried food, use oven baked instead, it is lower in fat.

19. Don't eat white refined foods like sugar, bread, rice, and flour. Use the unrefined brown foods.

20. Cut down on processed cereals, pies, cakes, pastries, biscuits, cookies, sweets, jam, chocolate, ice-cream, and soft drinks.

21. Don't eat food with preservatives or chemical coloring in them.

22. Don't eat sulphur dried fruits have the sun dried varieties from the health food shop.

23. Cut down on sauces, like mustard, pickles, Worcestershire sauce, curry, mayonnaise and salad dressing.

24. Eat as many raw vegetables, sprouted seeds, grains and legumes and fruit as you like. They are packed with vitamins and minerals and are the most

nutritious foods there are. Cooking destroys the enzymes and some of the vitamins in vegetables and fruit.

SOME BENEFITS OF EATING AND DRINKING CORRECTLY

- You will have more energy to spare and feel less fatigued.
- You will no longer need cups of coffee to keep you going.
- You won't have an energy lapse after lunch.
- When you eat better food your stress levels drop and you can relax easier.
- Your body will gradually normalize its weight and maintain that new weight.
- Exercising will be more enjoyable with your higher energy levels.
- Each change you can make to improve your eating habits for the good could add years to your life-span.
- Gradually as these positive good eating habits accumulate they build your new healthier body.

'Water is the only drink for a wise man'. (Thorau.)

CHAPTER ELEVEN:
MAKING THE CHANGE IN YOUR EATING HABITS

Many people say that changing is too difficult and they lack the will power to do it. That's why diets fail for a lot of people. Most diets require dramatic changes all at once or it's a waste of time. There are so many things you are not allowed to eat, then there's calorie counting and the cost can be prohibitive. Then as soon as you come off the diet you put on the weight again twice as fast. With correct eating you can eat as much as you want, you don't have to starve yourself to lose weight, you don't have to count calories. You may even find your shopping bill goes down as fresh food is often cheaper than packaged processed food.

Don't try to make drastic changes to your eating habits all at once, make the changes gradually. You are more likely to succeed if you take things slowly. The first week cut down on salt, eventually cutting it out all together. The next week cut down on fatty food and so on until you have made all the changes little by little. By the time you have slowly made your changes you will hardly have noticed it. We have learnt our present eating habits over a lifetime and those habits have become part of our lives, some of those habits may be hard to break. Habits can be changed though; you can learn to enjoy new and different ways of eating if you give yourself a chance. Don't be too hard on yourself if you slip up and fall back to old habits, just make up for it with your next meal of healthy food.

Here are a few self affirmations that may help you to visualize yourself eating properly and reaping the rewards. Repeat them to yourself when you feel your will power slipping a little.

Self Affirmations

- My food energizes me.
- I eat to improve myself.
- I energize my body with food.
- Food gives me energy.

- I am getting slimmer every day.
- I eat away the excess kilos.
- My food energy burns off the fat.
- I eat to be healthy.
- I have a right to good health.
- My body knows how to stay healthy.
- My food is my medicine.

WATER

Tap water contains many things that are bad for our health such as chlorine, rust, dirt, insecticides, pesticides, viruses and heavy metals like lead. Chlorine destroys vitamin E and C and these are essential for healthy hearts and the proper functioning of your cells and the circulation, as well as your ability to fight disease. Chlorine destroys all bacteria; it kills the friendly bacteria and enzymes in your digestive system so you do not get all the nutrition from your food due to mal-absorption. You feel constantly hungry and overeat, the result is more toxins than your body can get rid of and these are stored as fat.

Although rainwater doesn't have chlorine it contains many other nasty things. If you live in the city there is pollution from traffic emissions that fall in the form of acid rain. There are also pesticides, insecticides and bird droppings, dead insects and rotting foliage that harbour all sorts of fungi, viruses and bacteria. Even if you live in the country things are not much better.

Spring water has pesticides, insecticides, bacteria and viruses that filter down through the soil into the spring. There are also hard to metabolize heavy metals such as lead which your body must store as it cannot get rid of them. Too much lead can cause mental retardation in children and health problems in adults in the form of lead poisoning. The CSIRO found that home plumbing is often the source of excessive levels of lead. All these things pollute your body and hasten the process of secondary aging. The best water to drink is filtered water whether it is spring or tap water. Apart from water purifiers that are fitted to the kitchen sink, you can get filter tanks and jugs for drinking water that will filter out 99% of all impurities. They are a cheap alternative to expensive water purifiers. Many water authorities recommend fitting water purifiers to water tanks used for drinking water due to the toxins present in the water. Never drink distilled water as it is highly acidic and will leach minerals from your body, which could cause a mineral deficiency.

Whatever you decide to do, this is one change for the better you should do now don't put it off. It is probably the easiest change to make and the most beneficial.

FASTING FOR RAPID DE-TOXIFICATION

Fasting is abstaining from eating food for a period longer than you would normally between meals. Fluid must be taken during fasting as going without would seriously damage your health. When fasting is undertaken you should drink fruit and vegetable juice, warm purified water and herbal tea. Don't drink coffee, drinking chocolate, caffeinated tea, soft drinks or cordials; they will defeat the purpose of the fast by polluting your body.

A fast can last from a few hours up to 10 days, however if you intend to fast for more than 3 days you should do it under medical supervision. Fasting is a quick way to de-toxify your body, speed up weight loss and re-juvinate your body. It gives your body a chance to clear out all the accumulated rubbish and waste food in your digestive system and gives that system a well deserved rest. Because juices and herbal tea are very quickly and easily digested little energy is expended and your body has energy to spare for the important process of de-toxification of the body. If you fast for longer than 3 days your body will start to use up fat cells, the diseased, dying and dead cells and any other toxic waste that is available. If the fast is longer than 10 days the body will begin to use muscle tissue, since this is not desirable one would be well advised not to continue. Fasting for extreme lengths of time can lead to permanent damage to major organs and the autonomic nervous system. During a fast you don't use much energy for digestion so there is more energy available for de-toxification of the body and building of new cells which will proceed at a greatly accelerated rate during fasting. Fasting can help you live longer as well. Studies showed that the life of worms was prolonged to 50 times their normal life-span by fasting. Other studies have shown that the life-spans of rats were increased by 2 ½ times by fasting them every other day. People may not be able to increase their life-span quite so dramatically but fasting has long been an ancient method for healing ill health and prolonging life. Regular fasting was recommended by such great doctors of olden times as Galen and Hippocrates.

Note: If you have diabetes consult your doctor before undertaking a fast.

'Good health and good sense are the two blessings in life'. (Menander.)

CHAPTER: TWELVE
THE GLYCEMIC INDEX

GI stands for Glycemic Index. The GI is a ranking of carbohydrates on a scale from 0 to 100 according to the extent to which they raise blood sugar levels after eating, with sugar being the highest at 100.

More than 20% of Australians are obese and another 40% are overweight. We seem to be eating the same amount of fat over the last decade or so but we have seen a big increase in the amount of carbohydrates we eat, such as quick one minute breakfast oats, white refined bread and flours, cakes, burgers and biscuits. The more a food is processed the easier it is to digest and the quicker it is digested the sooner you feel hungry again and the more you tend to eat, these sorts of food are usually high GI foods. Low GI diets can prevent the most common diseases of affluence, such as coronary heart disease, diabetes (types 1 & 2) and obesity.

Everyone can use the GI index to maintain a normal blood sugar level. Higher than normal blood sugar can increase your risk of developing types 1 & 2 diabetes and heart disease. If you constantly eat high GI foods you very quickly become hungry again, this can trigger overeating and lead to weight gain. Every time you eat a high GI food your blood sugar level shoots up and your poor overworked pancreas releases insulin. People who develop diabetes cannot produce enough insulin or none at all. They also become insulin resistant, which means they cannot use the insulin in their blood to transport the glucose into the muscles where it is used for energy. This leads to organ damage like blood vessels, nervous system, heart attacks, kidney damage, blindness and loss of limbs. Generally the faster the food breaks down and is absorbed into the body the higher the Glycemic Index rating. When trying to lose weight or minimize the risk or manage diabetes, one should limit foods that have a high GI rating. By eating low GI foods you will maintain a steady normal blood sugar level and feel full up for longer.

Low GI diets are easy to apply; it doesn't mean you have to cut out a lot of foods. If you simply substitute low GI foods for high ones on average then you will have achieved a good balance between high and low GI foods. Just consider the high GI foods at each meal and substitute a low or intermediate one (e.g.: pasta or sweet potato instead of white potato. Apples, oranges and pears instead of tropical fruits.)

What is the significance of the GI index?
- Low GI means a smaller rise in blood glucose levels after meals.
- Low GI diets can help people lose weight.
- Low GI diets can improve the body's sensitivity to insulin.
- Low GI foods can help re-fuel carbohydrate stores after exercise.
- Low GI can improve diabetes control.
- Low GI can improve physical endurance.

How can you change over to a low GI diet? Use breakfast cereals based on oats (not instant oats these are high GI, use the old fashioned ones you have to cook), barley and bran. Use grainy breads made from whole seeds like Soy and Linseed bread or multigrain. Reduce the amount of white potato's you eat or cut them out completely, eat sweet potato instead (it's high in antioxidants). Eat lots of fresh fruit and vegetables (except white potato's & tropical fruits) check the list to see which ones are low GI, intermediate GI or high GI. Eat lots of salads; with a vinaigrette dressing (olive oil and Balsamic vinegar) vinegar helps to slow down the digestive process.

For people with diabetes a low GI diet can enhance their quality of life and help control that all important blood sugar level.

The GI rating sets glucose (sugar) at 100 and scores all other foods against that number.

Low GI Foods   **Below 55**
Intermediate GI Foods   **Between 55 and 70**

* Foods containing Fat in excess of National Heart Foundation guidelines

- **Low GI Food Below 55**

All bran	M 'n' Ms
Apple dried	Noodles 2 minute
Apple Muffin*	Noodles mung bean
Apple	Noodles rice
Apricot (dried)	Nutella
Apple juice	Oranges
Burgen soy-lin loaf	Orange juice
Burgen mixed grain loaf	Peaches
Black-eyed beans	Porridge
Barley pearled	Pasta Ravioli
Baked Beans	Pasta Egg Fettuccine
Buckwheat cooked	Pasta Spaghetti
Burgen ™ Fruit Loaf	Pasta Vermicelli
Bulgur (Burghul) cooked	Pear
Banana Cake	Plum
Butter Beans	Pumpernickel bread
Baked beans	Peas fresh
Chocolate white	Potato Crisps*
Chocolate pudding	Peanuts*
Chocolate mousse	Pea soup
Chocolate fudge cake	Peanuts roasted *
Chocolate butterscotch	Peas dried
Chicken nuggets	Party meat pies
Capellini pasta	Performax loaf
Carrot Cake	Pineapple juice
Carrots	Pinto beans
Chick Peas	Pizza supreme
Chocolate*	Ploughman's loaf
Custard	Pound cake
Cherries	Prunes
Cranberry juice	Ravioli pasta
Corn chips	Rice bran
Diet Soft Drink	Rolled oats
Doongara Rice	Romano beans
Diet Cordial	Soy & Linseed Bread
Fruit Loaf	Sweet potato
Fish Fingers	Swede
Fructose	Soya Beans
French vanilla cake	Sausages*
Fruit 'n' spice loaf	Snickers
Grapefruit	Sourdough rye loaf
Grapes green	Sourdough wheat loaf
Gluten free pasta	Soy milk

Grapefruit juice	Soy yogurt mango
Haricot Beans (navy beans)	Soya beans
Healthwise cereal	Soya beans canned
Hyfibe wholemeal loaf	Spaghetti white pasta
Ice cream low fat	Spaghetti wholemeal pasta
Kidney Beans	Spireli durum pasta
Kellogg's Guardian ™	Sponge cake
Kiwifruit fruit	Star pasta
Kellogg's All bran ™	Stoneground wholemeal flour
Komplete cereal	Strawberry jam
Kellogg's Special K ™	Sustagen milk chocolate
Lentils red, brown & green	Sustagen pudding
Lentil soup	Sustagen sports drink
Lactose	Tomatoes fresh
Linguine pasta thick	Tomatoes canned
Lima beans baby	Tortellini pasta
Milkshake low fat	Tomato soup
Milk	Vaalia yogurt
Milo	Vaalia yogurt no fat
Most Fruit and Vegetables	Vaalia pudding
Multigrain Bread	Vermicelli pasta
Milky bar	Weis mango fruitia
Multigrain Tip Top loaf	White Beans
Muesli toasted	Yakult probiotic
Mung beans	Yam
Marmalade	Yogurt low fat
Macaroni pasta	

- **Intermediate GI Food Between 55 and 70**

Arrowroot biscuits	Mars Bar *
Angel cake	Muesli Bar *
Apricot muffin	Nesquik Chocolate drink
Apricots canned	New potatoes canned
Apricots fresh	Nutri-grain cereal
Banana	Oat bran raw
Banana muffin	Oatmeal biscuit
Beetroot canned	Oatmeal
Black bean soup	Orange cordial
Blueberry muffin	Peach canned
Bran buds	Pizza cheese & tomato
Bran muffin	Popcorn
Breadfruit	Pineapple fresh
Breton wheat crackers	Pita Bread
Chocolate butterscotch muffins	Paw paw
Coca cola	Ploughman's wholemeal loaf
Condensed milk sweetened	Pop tarts double choc
Cornmeal (polenta)	Popcorn low fat
Couscous	Power bar chocolate
Croissant *	Quik chocolate drink
Crumpet	Rockmelon
Cordial	Rice Basmati
Digestive biscuit	Rice Arborio
Flaky pastry	Rice Doongara

Flan cake	Raisins
Froot loops	Ryvita
Frosties cereal	Rice vermicelli
Fruit cocktail canned	Rich tea biscuit
Fruit fingers banana	Riga sunflower & barley loaf
Fanta	Rye bread
Gnocchi	Ryvita crackers
Green pea soup	Semolina cooked
Greens pancakes	Shredded wheatmeal biscuit
Hamburger bun	Sucrose
Healthwise cereal	Sanitarium Wheet-Bix ™
Helgas classic seed loaf	Shortbread
Honey smacks cereal	Sweet Corn
Honey	Sao crackers
Ice cream full fat	Sultanas
Isostar sports drink	Shortbread biscuit
Jam apricot	Shredded wheat cereal
Just right cereal	Skittles
Just right just grains cereal	Spaghetti gluten free
Jatz Crackers	Split pea soup canned
Kudos Choc chip bar	Stoned wheat thins crackers
Kellogg's Sustain ™	Sustain bar
Kellogg's Nutrigrain ™	Sustain cereal
Life Savers ™	Sweet corn canned
Light rye loaf	Taco Shells
Linguine pasta thin	Tapioca steamed
Linseed rye loaf	Vaalia yogurt drink passion fruit
Macaroni	Vaalia yogurt passion fruit
Mango	Vitabrits cereal
Melba toast	Vitari frozen fruit
Milk arrowroot biscuit	Vogel's honey & oat loaf
Mini wheat's whole wheat cereal	Vogel's roggenbrot
Muesli bar with fruit	Weet-bix cereal
Muesli untoasted	White bread
Mini wheat's ™	Wholemeal bread

- **High GI Food Over 70**

Bagel	Lamingtons
Black rye loaf	Lebanese loaf
Bran flakes	Lucozade ™
Bread stuffing	Maltose
Buckwheat pancakes	Millet cooked
Burger rings	Mini wheat's blackcurrant cereal
Biscuits Morning Coffee	Morning coffee biscuit
Broad Beans	New potato
Cheerios cereal	Oat & Honey bake cereal
Glucose	Parsnips
Corn bran cereal	Pikelets
Corn chex cereal	Pontiac potato
Corn pasta	Premium soda crackers
Corn pops cereal	Pretzels
Corn thins	Puffed crispbread
Crispix cereal	Puffed wheat cereal

Crunchy nut bar	Pumpkin
Crunchy nut cereal	Real fruit bar
Cupcakes with icing	Rice broken white
Dark rye shinkenbrot loaf	Rice bubbles cereal
Dates dried	Rice cakes
Desiree potato	Rice chex cereal
Donut	Rice crispies
English muffin	Rice glutinous white
Fibre plus bar	Rice instant
Fortijuice summerfruits	Rice Jasmine
French baguette	Rice pelde brown
French fries	Rice sunbrown quick
Gatorade sports drink	Ris 'O' Mais Gluten free pasta
Glucose powder	Roll-ups
Gluten free loaf	Rice Calrose Long Grain
Gluten free multigrain	Rice Brown
Golden wheat's cereal	Rye Bread
Graham wafers	Scones
Grapenuts cereal	Sebago potato
Honey rice bubbles	Tapioca boiled
Instant potato	Team cereal
Jelly Beans	Tofu frozen dessert
Kellogg's Coco pops [TM]	Total cereal
Kellogg's Cornflakes [TM]	Twisties
Kellogg's Rice Bubbles [TM]	Vanilla wafer
Kellogg's Sultana Bran [TM]	Wheatbites cereal
K time bar	Wonder white high maize loaf
K time strawberry bar	Water Cracker
Kaiser roll	Waffles
Kavli crackers	White Potato
Kavil	Watermelon

Don't think you can't eat high GI foods at all though; the idea is to include a high GI food occasionally, the intermediate GI foods in moderation and mostly low GI foods.

Books about the Glycemic Index

- The New Glucose Revolution.

- The New Glucose Revolution: Life Plan

- The New Glucose Revolution: Top 100 Low GI Foods

- The New Glucose Revolution: Losing Weight

- The New Glucose Revolution: Sugar

- The New Glucose Revolution: People With Diabetes

- The New Glucose Revolution: Metabolic Syndrome And Your Heart

- The New Glucose Revolution: Peak Performance
- The New Glucose Revolution: Childhood Diabetes
- The New Glucose Revolution: Healthy Kids
- The New Glucose Revolution: GI Values

For more information on these books go to the website

http://www.glycemicindex.com/books-australia.htm

WEIGHT CHARTS

These charts are meant to be used as guidelines only.

IDEAL WEIGHT FOR MEN
SMALL FRAME

Ft - ins	cm	Small	Frame
		lbs	Kg
5.2	157.48	123 - 129	55.35 - 58.05
5.3	160.02	125 - 131	56.25 - 58.95
5.4	162.56	127- 133	57.15 - 59.85
5.5	165.10	129 - 135	58.05 - 60.75
5.6	167.64	131 - 137	58.95 - 61.65
5.7	170.18	133 - 140	59.85 - 63
5.8	172.72	135 - 143	60.75 - 64.35
5.9	175.26	137 - 146	61.65 - 65.70
5.10	177.78	139 - 149	62.55 – 67.05
5.11	180.34	141 - 152	63.45 – 68.40
6.0	182.88	144 - 155	64.80 – 69.75
6.1	185.42	147 - 159	66.15 – 71.55
6.2	187.96	150 - 163	67.50 – 73.35
6.3	190.50	153 - 167	68.85 – 75.15
6.4	193.04	157 - 171	70.65 – 76.95

IDEAL WEIGHT FOR MEN
MEDIUM FRAME

Ft - ins	cm	Medium	Frame
		lbs	Kg
5.2	157.48	126 - 136	56.70 – 61.20
5.3	160.02	128 - 138	57.60 – 62.10
5.4	162.56	130 - 140	58.50 – 63
5.5	165.10	132 - 143	59.40 – 64.35
5.6	167.64	134 - 146	60.30 – 65.70
5.7	170.18	137 - 149	61.65 – 67.05
5.8	172.72	140 - 152	63 – 68.40
5.9	175.26	143 - 155	64.35 – 69.75
5.10	177.78	146 - 158	65.70 – 71.10
5.11	180.34	149 - 161	67.05 – 72.45
6.0	182.88	152 - 165	68.40 – 74.25
6.1	185.42	155 - 169	69.75 – 76.05
6.2	187.96	159 - 173	71.55 – 77.85
6.3	190.50	162 - 177	72.90 – 79.65
6.4	193.04	166 - 182	74.70 – 81.90

IDEAL WEIGHT FOR MEN
LARGE FRAME

Ft - ins	cm	Large	Frame
		lbs	Kg
5.2	157.48	133 - 145	59.85 – 65.25
5.3	160.02	135 - 148	60.75 – 66.60
5.4	162.56	137 - 151	61.65 – 67.95
5.5	165.10	139 - 155	62.55 – 69.75
5.6	167.64	141 - 159	63.45 – 71.55
5.7	170.18	144 - 163	64.80 – 73.35
5.8	172.72	147 - 167	66.15 – 75.15
5.9	175.26	150 - 175	67.50 – 76.95
5.10	177.78	153 - 175	68.85 – 78.75
5.11	180.34	156 - 179	70.20 – 80.55
6.0	182.88	159 - 189	71.55 – 82.35
6.1	185.42	163 - 187	73.35 – 84.15
6.2	187.96	169 - 192	76.05 – 86.40
6.3	190.50	171 - 197	76.95 – 88.65
6.4	193.04	176 - 202	79.20 – 90.90

IDEAL WEIGHT FOR WOMEN
SMALL FRAME

Ft - ins	cm	Small	Frame
		lbs	Kg
4.10	147.32	99 - 108	44.55 – 48.60
4.11	149.86	100 - 110	45 – 49.50
5.0	152.40	101 - 112	45.45 – 50.40
5.1	154.94	103 - 115	46.35 – 51.75
5.2	157.45	105 - 118	47.25 – 53.10
5.3	160.02	108 - 121	48.60 – 54.45
5.4	162.56	111 - 125	49.95 – 56.25
5.5	165.10	114 - 127	51.30 – 57.15
5.6	167.64	117 - 130	52.65 – 58.50
5.7	170.18	120 - 133	54 – 59.85
5.8	172.72	123 - 136	55.35 – 61.20
5.9	175.26	126 - 139	56.70 – 62.55
5.10	177.78	129 - 142	58.05 – 63.90
5.11	180.34	132 - 145	59.40 – 65.25
6.0	193.04	135 - 148	60.75 – 66.60

IDEAL WEIGHT FOR WOMEN
MEDIUM FRAME

Ft - ins	cm	Medium	Frame
		lbs	Kg
4.10	147.32	106 - 118	47.70 – 53.10
4.11	149.86	108 - 120	48.60 – 54
5.0	152.40	110 - 123	49.50 – 55.35
5.1	154.94	112 - 126	50.40 – 56.70
5.2	157.45	115 - 129	51.75 – 58.05
5.3	160.02	118 - 132	53.1059.40
5.4	162.56	121 - 135	54.45 – 60.75
5.5	165.10	124 - 138	55.80 – 62.10
5.6	167.64	127 - 141	57.15 – 63.45
5.7	170.18	130 - 144	58.50 – 64.80
5.8	172.72	133 - 147	59.85 – 66.15
5.9	175.26	136 - 150	61.20 – 67.50
5.10	177.78	139 - 153	62.55 – 68.85
5.11	180.34	142 –156	63.90 – 70.20
6.0	193.04	145 - 159	65.25 – 71.55

IDEAL WEIGHT FOR WOMEN
HEAVY FRAME

Ft - ins	cm	Heavy	Frame
		lbs	Kg
4.10	147.32	115 - 128	51.75 – 57.60
4.11	149.86	117 - 131	52.65 – 58.95
5.0	152.40	119 - 134	53.55 – 60.30
5.1	154.94	122 – 137	54.90 – 61.65
5.2	157.45	125 - 140	56.25 – 63
5.3	160.02	128 - 144	57.60 – 64.80
5.4	162.56	131 - 148	58.95 – 66.60
5.5	165.10	134 - 152	60.30 – 68.40
5.6	167.64	137 -156	61.65 – 70.20
5.7	170.18	140 - 160	63 – 72
5.8	172.72	143 - 164	64.35 – 73.80
5.9	175.26	146 - 167	65.70 – 75.15
5.10	177.78	149 - 170	67.05 – 76.50
5.11	180.34	152 - 173	68.40 – 77.85
6.0	193.04	155 - 176	69.75 – 79.20

FOOD PYRAMID

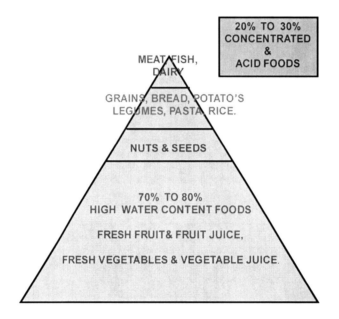

20% TO 30%
CONCENTRATED
&
ACID FOODS

MEAT, FISH,
DAIRY

GRAINS, BREAD, POTATO'S
LEGUMES, PASTA, RICE.

NUTS & SEEDS

70% TO 80%
HIGH WATER CONTENT FOODS

FRESH FRUIT& FRUIT JUICE,

FRESH VEGETABLES & VEGETABLE JUICE.

THE HUMAN BODY IS MADE UP OF 30% CONCENTRATED
SUBSTANCES LIKE BONES, MUSCLES, LIGAMENTS & TENDONS.

THE OTHER 70% IS WATER CONTENT BLOOD & INTERSTITIAL
FLUIDS.

THREE WEEKS MEAL PLANNER

All these lunch & dinner meals can have meat or fish added if they don't already have them included in the recipe. Vegetarians can substitute non animal products.

WEEK ONE

DAY	BREAKFAST	SNACK	LUNCH	SNACK	DINNER	SUPPER
MONDAY	Toast Multigrain bread & fruit juice	Raw vegetable Carrot & celery	Tunisian tuna salad	Fruit	Leek, proscuitto & rice frittata	Low fat yogurt
TUESDAY	Cereal All Bran & vegetable juice	Fruit Apple & banana	Tabbouleh salad	Crackers & dip	Fish with beans & tomato	Peanut sandwich
WEDNESDAY	Fruit Banana & Apple & vegetable juice	Low fat yogurt	Pumpkin soup	Fruit	Capsicum casserole	Apple muffin
THURSDAY	Porridge Fruit juice	Fruit orange & apple	Salad with everything	Raw vegetable	Mixed vegetable chow mien	Low fat muesli bar
FRIDAY	Cereal Special K fruit juice	Raw vegetable tomato celery	Chick pea soup	Low fat yogurt	Pepperoni risotto	Crackers & cheese
SATURDAY	Toast multigrain bread & vegetable juice	Fruit banana & apple	Tandoori chicken salad	Raw vegetable	Layered rice cake With salmon or tuna	Apple muffin
SUNDAY	Porridge fruit juice	Apple muffin	Beef soup	Fruit	Italian - Style Chicken	Nutella sandwich

WEEK TWO

DAY	BREAKFAST	SNACK	LUNCH	SNACK	DINNER	SUPPER
MONDAY	Toast Multigrain bread & fruit juice	Raw vegetable Carrot & celery	Caesar Salad	Fruit	Nutty cheese & rice frittata	Low fat yogurt
TUESDAY	Cereal All Bran & vegetable juice	Fruit Apple & banana	Mulligatawny soup	Crackers & dip	Char grilled salmon and herb sauce	Peanut sandwich
WEDNESDAY	Fruit Banana & Apple & vegetable juice	Low fat yogurt	Waldorf salad	Fruit	Gardeners pie	Apple muffin
THURSDAY	Porridge Fruit juice	Fruit orange & apple	Tomato & lentil soup	Raw vegetable	Italian style chicken	Low fat muesli bar
FRIDAY	Cereal Special K fruit juice	Raw vegetable tomato celery	Salade Nicoise	Low fat yogurt	Grilled vegetable flan	Crackers & cheese
SATURDAY	Toast multigrain bread & vegetable juice	Fruit banana & apple	Black eyed bean soup	Raw vegetable	Onion spinach & cheese frittata	Apple muffin
SUNDAY	Porridge fruit juice	Apple muffin	Tunisian tuna salad	Fruit	Wholemeal lentil lasagna	Nutella Sandwich

WEEK THREE

DAY	BREAKFAST	SNACK	LUNCH	SNACK	DINNER	SUPPER
MONDAY	Toast Multigrain bread & fruit juice	Raw vegetable Carrot & celery	Caesar Salad	Fruit	Nutty Cheese & Rice Frittata	Low fat yogurt
TUESDAY	Cereal All Bran & vegetable juice	Fruit Apple & banana	Mulligatawny soup	Crackers & dip	Gardeners Pie	Peanut sandwich
WEDNESDAY	Fruit Banana & Apple & vegetable juice	Low fat yogurt	Waldorf salad	Fruit	Grilled Vegetable Flan	Nutella sandwich
THURSDAY	Porridge Fruit juice	Fruit orange & apple	Pumpkin soup	Raw vegetable	Wholemeal Lentil Lasagna	Low fat muesli bar
FRIDAY	Cereal Special K fruit juice	Raw vegetable tomato celery	Salade Nicoise	Low fat yogurt	Fish With Beans & Tomatoes	Crackers & cheese
SATURDAY	Toast multigrain bread & vegetable juice	Fruit banana & apple	Beef soup	Raw vegetable	Mixed Vegetable Chow Mien	Apple muffin
SUNDAY	Porridge fruit juice	Apple muffin	Tunisian tuna salad	Fruit	Layered Rice Cake With Salmon Or Tuna	Nutella sandwich

There are soups, salads & dinner recipes to choose from.

If you usually eat your main meal in the middle of the day these planners can be altered to suit. If you don't like or can't get some of the ingredients in the recipes simply substitute something else or leave it out altogether. You can substitute meat for some of the vegetarian ingredients the recipes are designed to be flexible.

RECIPES

SALADS:

Caesar Salad:

Serves 4

7 slices multigrain bread

2 tablespoons light olive oil

100g parmesan cheese

1 large cos lettuce

5 whole canned anchovy fillets, drained, & halved lengthways

Caesar Dressing

1 egg

2 tablespoons lemon juice

½ teaspoon Dijon mustard

5 whole canned anchovy fillets, drained

¾ cup (180 ml) light olive oil

Caesar Salad: Method

Cut off crusts; cut bread into small cubes. Heat the oil in large pan; fry bread until brown & crisp. Drain croutons on absorbent paper. Use a vegetable peeler to shave parmesan into long thin pieces.

Combine torn lettuce leaves with half of the croutons, half the anchovies & half the cheese in a large bowl; add half of the dressing & mix well. Sprinkle the remaining croutons, anchovies & cheese over the salad; Drizzle the remaining dressing over the salad. Caesar dressing put all ingredients except oil into a blender & blend until smooth, while still blending add oil until dressing thickens.

Waldorf Salad:

Serves 4

4 medium (600g) apples

¼ cup (60 ml) lemon juice

5 trimmed celery sticks

1 cup (120g) coarsely chopped walnuts

Mayonnaise:

2 egg yolks

2 teaspoons lemon juice

1 teaspoon Dijon mustard

¼ cup (180 ml) olive oil

1 tablespoon warm water

Waldorf Salad: Method:

Core & coarsely chop apples. Combine apples & lemon juice in a bowl.

Coarsely chop celery.

Combine apple, celery & walnuts in a bowl with mayonnaise. Serve salad on a bed of lettuce if desired.

Mayonnaise: Method

Blend egg yolks, lemon juice & mustard until smooth add oil & water slowly while still blending until mayonnaise thickens.

Tabbouleh Salad:

3 medium (570g) tomatoes

½ cup (80g) burghul

5 cups tightly packed fresh parsley

1 medium (170g) red onion

1 cup tightly packed fresh mint leaves

¼ cup (60 ml) lemon juice

¼ cup (60 ml) olive oil

Method:

Chop tomatoes finely, place tomatoes on top of burghul in a bowl, cover; refrigerate for 2 hours or until burghul is soft.

Meanwhile chop parsley & mint coarsely, chop onion finely .

Combine all ingredients together in a bowl.

Salad With Everything:

Serves 4

4 medium tomatoes

4 sticks of celery

1 medium capsicum

6 medium mushrooms

1 medium zucchini

1 medium cucumber

6 spring onions

6 medium radishes

½ cup of parsley

½ cup of mint leaves

Salad With Everything: Vinaigrette Dressing:

¼ cup of Balsamic vinegar

¼ cup of olive oil

Decoration: (Optional)

2 Calendula flowers

8 Nasturtium flowers

Salad With Everything : Method:

Chop all ingredients coarsely and mix in a bowl .

Vinaigrette Dressing: Method

Mix Balsamic vinegar and olive oil together in bottle with lid, shake vigorously before pouring onto salad

Decoration:

Pull off Calendula petals and sprinkle over the salad.

Place Nasturtium flowers around the edges of the salad.

These flowers can be eaten as part of the salad.

Other flowers maybe used as well.

(See section on edible flowers)

Tunisian Tuna Salad:

Serves 4

2 hard boiled eggs

1 medium 200g green capsicum
 chopped finely

2 medium (380g) tomatoes chopped finely

4 spring onions finely chopped

2 large canned anchovy fillets chopped finely

10 seeded green or black olives chopped finely

2 red chillies, seeded & chopped finely

2 teaspoons fresh mint chopped finely

185g can of tuna, drained & flaked

1 tablespoon baby capers, drained.

1 teaspoon caraway seeds

1 tablespoon lemon juice

2 table spoons red wine vinegar

Harissa-Style Dressing

2 tablespoons olive oil

1 clove of garlic, crushed

1 teaspoon coriander seeds

Method:

Shell eggs & chop finely. Combine eggs with all the ingredients in a bowl; drizzle dressing over salad, mixed to combine.

Harissa-Style Dressing.

Heat the oil in a pan, add crushed garlic & seeds; cook, stirring until fragrant. Stir in lemon juice & vinegar

Tandoori Chicken Salad

Serves 4

500g Chicken tenderloins halved lengthways with skin removed

2 tablespoons tandoori paste

1 cos lettuce

1 medium mango (430g) sliced thinly

2 celery sticks sliced thinly

1 cucumber sliced thinly

1 small red onion (100g) sliced thinly

2 tablespoons fresh mint leaves

2 tablespoons unsalted peanuts

Yogurt Mint Dressing:

½ cup low fat yogurt

2 tablespoons water

½ teaspoon tandoori paste

1 pinch of ground cumin

1 small clove of garlic, crushed

1 tablespoon finely chopped fresh mint

Tandoori Chicken Salad: Method:

Combine chicken & tandoori paste in a bowl. Cook chicken in oiled frying pan until brown all over & cooked through.

Combine torn lettuce leaves in a bowl with other ingredients. Top with chicken, drizzle with dressing. Sprinkle with mint leaves & nuts.

Yogurt Dressing:

Blend ingredients until combined.

SOUPS:

Mulligatawny Soup:

Serves 6 to 8

30g of butter or margarine

1 small leek (200g) sliced

1 stick of celery finely chopped

1 medium carrot finely chopped

2 tablespoons Madras curry paste

2 cloves garlic, crushed

2 teaspoons grated fresh ginger

½ cup (100g) Arborio rice

1 ½ cups (375 ml) coconut milk

1 medium apple, grated

2 tablespoons lime juice

2 tablespoons chopped fresh coriander

Chicken Stock:

1.2 kg chicken

5 litres (20 cups) water

15 black peppercorns

1 large (200g) onion, quartered

1 large (180g) carrot, chopped

1 stick celery, chopped

4 sprigs fresh parsley

2 bay leaves

Mulligatawny Soup: Method:

Heat butter or margarine in a pan, add leek, celery, carrot & curry paste, cook stirring until leek is soft. Add ginger, garlic & rice. Cook stirring until fragrant. Add chicken stock, simmer uncovered 10 minutes, add coconut milk apple and chicken (from stock) simmer for 5 minutes. Just before serving add lime juice and coriander.

Chicken Stock:

Combine all ingredients in a pot simmer uncovered 1 ½ hours. Remove chicken, strain stock into a bowl discard vegetable mixture. Return chicken to stock leave to cool in refrigerator. When cold skim off fat , remove chicken from stock & remove meat from chicken bones. Chop up chicken meat & return to stock. Stock needs to be done well in advance or the day before.

Pumpkin Soup:

500g pumpkin

1 medium sweet potato finely chopped

¼ teaspoon of ground turmeric

¼ teaspoon garam masala

2 tablespoons water

1 medium leek chopped

1 stick of celery

1 large vegetable stock cube

Pumpkin Soup

2 cups (500 ml) extra water

2 tablespoons fresh chopped parsley

Pumpkin Soup: Method:

Cut pumpkin into small cubes cook ½ the pumpkin with sweet potato, drain & mash well. Add spices to a dry pan cook till fragrant. Add water, leek and celery cook until leek is soft. Add chopped raw pumpkin stock cube, remainder of water & mashed vegetable to the pan. Boil then simmer until pumpkin is soft, stir in parsley, serve with

Pumpkin Soup: Method:

toast or bread rolls.

Black-eyed Bean Soup:

1 cup (200g) dried black-eyed beans

1 tablespoon reduced-fat margarine

2 medium onions (300g) chopped finely

2 medium carrots (240g) chopped finely

1 small sweet potato (250g) chopped finely

1 medium turnip (125g) chopped finely

2 sticks of celery chopped finely

2 medium zucchini chopped finely

4 medium tomatoes chopped finely

2 cups (500 ml) water

1 large vegetable stock cube

2 teaspoons tomato paste

Black-eyed Bean Soup: Method:

Cover beans with cold water, leave overnight. Drain beans next day, cook onions, carrots & sweet potato in margarine 5 minutes. Add beans, zucchini, tomatoes water, stock cube & paste. Simmer for 45 minutes or until beans are tender. Serve with toast or bread rolls.

Beef Soup:

375g beef round steak, sliced thinly

1 tablespoon dry red wine

3 cups (750 ml) water

3 cups (750 ml) beef stock

6 small onions chopped finely

2 cloves garlic thinly sliced

3 fresh coriander roots

2 tablespoons light soy sauce

2 teaspoons brown sugar

1 red chillie chopped finely

425g button mushrooms

¼ cup (60 ml) lime juice

1 tablespoon finely chopped coriander leaves

Beef Soup: Method:

Combine beef & wine in a bowl cover & let stand for 15 minutes. Combine water, beef stock, onion, garlic, coriander roots, soy sauce, sugar & half the in a pan. Bring to the boil; simmer uncovered 15 minutes. Strain the soup return strained soup to the pan discard strained mixture. Before serving bring soup to the boil; add beef , mushrooms, remaining chillie & lime juice, simmer for 5 minutes, finally add coriander l eaves.

Serve with toast or bread rolls.

Tomato & Lentil Soup:

1 large onion

1 810g can or fresh tomatoes

125g red lentils

2 cups of vegetable stock

Fresh basil leaves

Tomatoe & Lentil Soup: Method:

Finely chop the onion simmer it until soft in a little water. Chop & add tomato. Add lentils & stock , bring to boil & simmer 30 minutes. Blend the soup until smooth chop basil finely & add. Reheat & serve with toast or bread rolls.

Chickpea Soup:

1 table spoon of water

1 large red onion chopped finely

2 cloves of garlic crushed

1 teaspoon ground cumin

1 teaspoon ground turmeric

1 teaspoon ground sweet paprika

½ teaspoon ground cinnamon

2 x 425g cans of chickpeas, rinsed & drained

300g can red kidney beans, rinsed & drained

½ cup (100g) red lentils

1.25 litres (5 cups) vegetable stock

¼ cup (60 ml) lemon juice

1/3 cup of chopped fresh mint leaves

1 bunch of spinach chopped

Chickpea Soup: Method:

Combine water, onion, garlic & spices in a pan cook until onion is soft. Add peas, beans, lentils, stock, lemon juice & mint simmer, covered, 20 minutes, stir occasionally until lentils are soft. Stir in spinach and simmer uncovered 5 minutes. Serve with toast or bread rolls.

DINNERS:

Char Grilled Salmon & Limes:

Serves 4

4 small salmon fillets

¼ cup (85g) lime marmalade

1 tablespoon rice vinegar

1 teaspoon grated fresh ginger

3 medium limes (240g) sliced thickly

Creamy Herb Sauce:

½ cup low fat yogurt (140g)

2 teaspoon finely chopped fresh mint

1 teaspoon finely chopped fresh dill

Char Grilled Salmon & Limes: Method:

Brush salmon with combined marmalade, vinegar, and ginger. Cook salmon & lime slices on heated oiled grill or barbecue until salmon is browned on both sides and cooked as desired & lime slices are browned on both sides. Serve salmon & lime with creamy herb sauce & a side salad of your choice.

Creamy Herb Sauce: Method:

Combine ingredients with a blender until smooth & creamy texture.

Gardeners Pie (Vegetarian Shepherds Pie)

Minced meat may be added)

1 cup brown lentils

1 teaspoon onion powder

1 tablespoon olive oil or vegetable stock

½ teaspoon oregano

3 tablespoon tomato paste

2 ½ cups sweet potato

Gardeners Pie: Method:

Boil in water then simmer the onion powder &

1 large onion chopped finely

1 clove garlic, crushed

1 cup mushrooms, sliced

1 stick celery, sliced

1 carrot finely sliced

½ cup broccoli finely chopped

1 tablespoon vegemite

1 tablespoon soy sauce

¾ cup vegetable stock

1 teaspoon mixed herbs

lentils until soft about 15 minutes then drain. Heat oil or stock in a pan & sauté onion garlic & mushrooms for 5 minutes. Add remaining vegetables & sauté 5 minutes. Add lentils, vegemite, soy sauce, vegetable stock, herbs & tomato paste. Stir over heat until combined then simmer for 5 minutes. Mixture should be fairly thick. Boil and mash sweet potatoes. Turn the filling into a deep dish top with mashed potato, bake in a hot oven for 15 minutes (220 degrees).

Nutty Cheese & Rice Frittata:

Serves 4 to 6

1 tablespoon light olive oil

2 chopped bacon rashers

1 medium (150g) onion, sliced

2 medium (240g) zucchini, sliced

1 clove garlic, crushed

½ teaspoon chopped fresh rosemary

6 eggs lightly beaten

1 cup cooked rice (Arborio, Basmati or Doongara

½ cup (60g) grated cheese, low fat

¼ cup (40g) pine nuts

Nutty Cheese & Rice Frittata: Method:

Crack eggs into a bowl, whisk till yolk and white are well combined. Put bacon, onion, zucchini, garlic, rosemary, rice and pine nuts into egg mixture and combine well.

Pour mixture into a frying pan and cook over a medium heat. To test whether it is done on the underside lift one edge carefully, if it is brown a little it is done. Sprinkle cheese on top of the frittata and place frying pan under the grill until golden brown.

Grilled Vegetable Flan:

Serves 4 to 6

2 cups of cooked brown rice

1 egg lightly beaten

½ cup (40g) grated parmesan cheese

2 medium (400g) red capsicum

4 medium (480g) zucchini

1 tablespoon olive oil

2 tablespoons pesto

2 eggs extra, lightly beaten

½ cup (125 ml) cream

Grilled Vegetable Flan: Method:

Process half the rice until finely chopped, combine processed rice with remaining rice, egg & cheese in a bowl mix well. Press rice mixture over the base & sides of a greased flan dish. Quarter capsicums & remove seeds & membranes, grill skin side up until skin blisters & blackens. Peel off skins and cut into strips, cut zucchinis into lengthways strips oil and grill until brown on both sides. Spread pesto over rice base & top with peppers & zucchini. Pour combined extra eggs & cream over vegetables. Bake uncovered in a moderate oven (180 degrees) for 35 minutes or until set.

Italian-Style Chicken:

Serves 4

4 chicken thighs (640g), skin removed

1 large brown onion (200g), chopped finely

2 cloves garlic, crushed

½ cup (125 ml) chicken stock

2 x 400g cans of tomatoes or 4 medium fresh tomatoes

2 tablespoons tomato paste

1 teaspoon brown sugar

2 tablespoons red wine vinegar

500g button mushrooms

2 teaspoons finely chopped fresh oregano

8 small zucchini (720) halved lengthways

Italian Style Chicken: Method:

Cook the chicken in a frying pan till both sides are brown, remove chicken from pan & drain fat on paper towel. Cook onion, garlic & chicken stock in the same frying pan for 5 minutes until onion is soft & liquid has evaporated. Return chicken to the pan with chopped tomatoes, paste, sugar, vinegar, mushroom & oregano simmer covered 1 hour. Remove the lid & simmer for 15 minutes till chicken is tender and sauce has thickened.

Meanwhile coat zucchini halves with olive oil & grill or barbecue until brown on both sides. Serve chicken mixture with char-grilled zucchini.

Onion Spinach & Cheese Frittata:

Serves 4

1 teaspoon of olive oil

3 medium brown onions(450g) sliced thinly

2 cloves of garlic, crushed

100g spinach leaves chopped finely

4 eggs beaten lightly

60g low fat grated cheddar cheese

1/3 cup (65g) low fat ricotta cheese

1 tablespoon finely grated parmesan cheese

1 tablespoon finely chopped fresh basil

1 tablespoon finely chopped fresh sage

Onion Spinach & Cheese Frittata: Method:

Heat the oil in a pan cook covered onion & garlic until very soft about 20 minutes. Add spinach stir until wilted. Combine onion mixture with eggs, cheeses & herbs in a bowl mix well. Pour egg mixture into oiled frying pan, cook over low heat for 10 minutes or until center begins to set. Place under a grill until frittata is set & top is browned lightly. Sprinkle a little extra grated cheese over the top before serving.

Wholemeal Lentil Lasagna:

Olive oil spray

1 ½ cups (300g) brown lentils

1 teaspoon olive oil

2 cloves garlic, crushed

1 medium (150g) onion, chopped

200g button mushrooms, sliced

1 medium (120g) zucchini, chopped

1 teaspoon garam masala

2 teaspoons ground cumin

6 instant wholemeal lasagna sheets

2 cups (400g) low fat ricotta cheese

¼ cup (15g) stale brown breadcrumbs

½ cup (50g) grated low fat mozzarella cheese

1 tablespoon chopped fresh parsley

Wholemeal Lentil Lasagna: Method:

Coat a large ovenproof dish or metal cake dish with olive oil spray. Boil lentils in a pan until tender (15 minutes). Heat the oil in a pan and add onion & garlic cook until soft, add capsicum, mushrooms, zucchini & spices cook until tender, stir in the lentils. Cover base of the prepared dish with 3 sheets of lasagna, spread with half the lentil mixture, then half the ricotta cheese. Repeat with remaining lasagna sheets , lentil mixture & ricotta cheese. Sprinkle with combined bread crumbs, mozzarella cheese & parsley. Bake uncovered in a moderate oven about 45 minutes until top is brown.

Leek, Prosciutto & Rice Frittata:

Serves 4 to 6

1 tablespoon olive oil

2 medium leeks (700g), chopped

3 slices prosciutto, chopped

7 eggs, lightly beaten

¼ cup (20g) grated parmesan cheese

½ cup skim milk or soy milk

1 cup cooked rice (Arborio, Basmati or Doongara

¼ cup chopped fresh chives

Leek, Prosciutto & Rice Frittata: Method:

Grease a deep 19 cm square cake pan. Heat oil in a frying pan, add leeks & prosciutto cook until leeks are soft. Combine leek mixture with remaining ingredients in a bowl; mix well. Pour the mixture into prepared cake pan, bake uncovered in a moderate oven about 35 minutes until lightly browned & set.

Fish With Beans & Tomato:

Serves 4

12 medium tomatoes halved

2 teaspoons olive oil

1 tablespoon brown sugar

2 tablespoons balsamic vinegar

2 cloves garlic, crushed

1 teaspoon salt

½ teaspoon cracked black pepper

350g baby green beans

4 fish fillets

Fish With Beans & Tomato:

10 fresh basil leaves, chopped

Fish With Beans & Tomato:Method:

Preheat the oven to hot. Combine tomato, oil, sugar, vinegar, garlic, salt & pepper in a large baking dish. Roast uncovered in a hot oven about 35 minutes until tomato is soft. Meanwhile boil steam or microwave beans until tender. Cook fish on an oiled grill or barbecue until brown both sides & just cooked through. Stir basil into tomato mixture, serve with fish & beans.

Capsicum With Zucchini & Beans:

Serves 4

½ cup (100g) dried borlotti beans

4 medium (800g) red capsicums

4 medium (480g) zucchini, chopped

4 baby onions, quartered

200g green beans, halved

300g can chickpeas, rinsed, drained

¼ cup (20g) flaked parmesan cheese

Tomato Sauce:

2 x 400g cans tomatoes

1 tablespoon balsamic vinegar

!/2 teaspoon sugar

¼ cup shredded fresh basil leaves

Capsicum With Zucchini & Beans: Method:

Soak borlotti beans overnight covered.

Drain beans, boil for 20 minutes until tender, drain. Halve the capsicums lengthways, remove seeds & membranes. Place in a shallow oven proof dish cut side up. Combine borlotti beans, zucchini, green beans & chickpeas in a bowl, mix well. Spoon mixture into capsicums; pour tomato sauce over them. Bake covered in a moderate oven 1 hour, remove cover bake about 15 minutes until capsicums are tender. Serve topped with parmesan cheese,

Tomato Sauce:

Combine crushed tomatoes with vinegar & sugar in a pan, simmer uncovered for 5 minutes until sauce is slightly thickened, stir in basil.

Pepperoni Risotto:

Serves 4

150g green beans, halved

1.5 litres (6 cups) Chicken stock

2 tablespoons tomato paste

1 tablespoon olive oil

20g butter or margarine

1 large (200g) onion, chopped

1 medium (200g) red capsicum, chopped

2 cups (400g) Arborio rice

200g pepperoni, sliced

1/3 cup (50g) stuffed green olives

Pepperoni Risotto: Method:

Add beans to boiling water , drain immediately, rinse under cold water, drain. Combine stock & paste in a pan, bring to the boil, cover & keep hot. Heat oil & butter or margarine in a pan, add onion & pepper, cook until onion is soft. Stir in rice then 2/3 of a cup (160 ml) of boiling stock mixture, cook over a low heat until liquid is absorbed. Continue adding stock mixture gradually , until absorbed before adding more. Total cooking time about 35 minutes or until rice is tender. Stir in pepperoni & beans & stir until hot.

Mixed Vegetable Chow Mien:

5 Mushrooms

350g packet thin fresh egg noodles

1 teaspoon olive oil

olive oil spray

3 cloves garlic, crushed

1 tablespoon grated fresh ginger

1 small fresh red chilli, chopped finely

1 medium (120g) carrot sliced

2 sticks of celery, sliced

125g snow peas, sliced

1 small (400g) Chinese cabbage shredded

425g can baby corn drained & sliced

2 teaspoons (60 ml) cornflour

¼ cup water

1 cup (250 ml) vegetable stock

Mixed Vegetable Chow Mien:

2 teaspoons soy sauce

1 tablespoon hoi sin sauce

6 spring onions, sliced

Mixed Vegetable Chow Mien: Method:

Place mushrooms in a bowl & cover with boiling water let them stand for 20 minutes. Drain mushrooms & chop finely. Rinse noodles under cold water, drain. Combine noodles with oil in a bowl. Heat wok or deep frying pan coat with spray oil, add noodles, stir fry 2 minutes then remove from pan. Heat the same wok or fry pan coat with oil spray, add garlic, ginger, chilli, mushrooms, carrot & celery, stir fry until carrot is just tender. Add snow peas, cabbage & corn, stir fry until cabbage has wilted. Add blended cornflour & water, stock & sauces, stir over heat until sauce boils and thickens slightly. Add noodles & onions stir until heated through.

Layered Rice Cake:

Serves 6

415g can of salmon, drained & flaked

2 cups cooked rice (Arborio, Basmati or Doongara

2 spring onions, chopped

2 eggs, lightly beaten

1 teaspoon grated lemon rind

Spinach Layer:

1 tablespoon olive oil

1 medium (150g) onion, chopped

1 clove garlic, crushed

250g chopped spinach, frozen or fresh

2 cups cooked rice (Arborio, Basmati or Doongara

2 eggs, lightly beaten

Cheese Herb Layer:

2 cups cooked rice (Arborio, Basmati or Doongara

Layered Rice Cake:

1 tablespoon chopped fresh basil

½ cup (40g) grated parmesan cheese

2 eggs, lightly beaten

Layered Rice Cake: Method:

Combine salmon, rice, spring onions, eggs & lemon rind in a bowl; mix well. Spread mixture over the base of a greased spring form tin. Top with spinach layer, then cheese & herb layer. Bake uncovered in a moderate oven for 45 minutes until set. Stand for 10 minutes before slicing. Serve with mayonnaise.

Spinach Layer:

Heat oil in a pan, add onion, garlic & spinach, cook until liquid has evaporated, cool. Combine spinach mixture with rice & eggs in a bowl; mix well.

Cheese & Herb Layer:

Combine all ingredients in a bowl; mix well.

Roasted Capsicum With Tomato & Rice:

Serves 4 to 6

4 large (1.4k) red capsicums, halved lengthways

¼ cup (60 ml) olive oil

1 medium (150g) onion, chopped

1 clove garlic, crushed

1 ½ cups cooked Basmati rice

1 /3 cup dry white wine

425g can tomatoes

2 cups (500 ml) chicken stock

Roasted Capsicum With Tomato & Rice: Method:

Remove seeds & membranes from capsicums, brush skins of capsicums with olive oil, place them on an oven tray, bake uncovered in a moderate oven 15 minutes. Heat remaining oil in a pan, add onion, garlic & cooked rice, cook until onion is soft. Add wine cook until wine is absorbed. Stir in crushed tomatoes add one cup of chicken stock & paste cook until piqued

1 tablespoon tomato paste

3 small (270g) zucchini, chopped

2 (120g) finger eggplants, chopped

125g feta cheese, crumbled

1 teaspoon fresh chopped oregano

1 teaspoon fresh chopped basil

2 teaspoons fresh chopped parsley

is absorbed. Stir in remaining stock, zucchini & eggplants; cook covered over a low heat until liquid is absorbed & vegetables are tender, stir occasionally. Spoon mixture into roasted capsicums, sprinkle with cheese & herbs. Bake uncovered in a moderate oven for 20 minutes or until cheese has melted.

More Easy Recipes To Cook In Minutes

Carrot & Leek Soup:

2 medium leeks, chopped

4 small carrots, chopped

150 ml cows milk or soy milk

seasoning to taste

Method:

Cook the vegetables in 300 ml water for 10 to 15 minutes until tender. Mash or liquidize, return to the pan, add the milk, salt & pepper to taste. Bring to the boil, simmer for 2 to 3 minutes. Pour the soup into containers and freeze. To serve thaw and heat

Tomato Soup:

8 large tomato's, sliced

2 large onions, sliced

2 carrots diced

5 sticks of celery, chopped

60 gm low fat margarine

2 litres of chicken stock

Salt to taste

Method:

Melt the margarine in a large pot, add vegetables & stock, simmer for 2 ½ hrs.

Mash or liquidize, season to taste. Pour the soup into containers and freeze. To serve thaw and heat

Easy Salad:

1 tomato, sliced in rounds

1 carrot, cut into small slivers

whole lettuce leaf

cucumber, sliced on the diagonal

radish, chopped

celery chopped into small pieces

sprouts

edible flowers

seasoning to taste

Method:

Place lettuce leaf on plate as a bed. Arrange other ingredients on the lettuce leaf decorate with edible flowers. Season to taste.

Steak & Kidney Stew:

Fillet of lean topside steak

6 lambs kidneys

1 large carrot, chopped

6 large Brussels sprouts, cut in halves

1 cup of peas

½ cup of broad beans

Steak & Kidney Stew:

1 medium onion, chopped

1 meat stock cube

seasoning to taste

Method:

Cut the steak & kidneys into small pieces. Put all the ingredients into a stock pot with sufficient water to cover them & bring to the boil, simmer for 3 hrs. Pour the stew into containers and freeze. To serve thaw and heat

Curried Rice Salad:

225 gm Arborio or Basmati rice

1 stick celery, chopped

1 tomato, chopped

1 green capsicum, chopped

1 grated carrot

2 tablespoons water

curry powder to taste 1-3 teaspoons

Method:

Cook rice till tender, drain. Stir curry powder and water together. Pour over the rice while still warm & mix. Add the salad when rice has cooled and mix together.

Stir Fry Chicken, Nuts & Vegetables:

500gm chicken breasts

½ teaspoon five spice powder

½ teaspoon salt to taste

200gm nuts

1 cup snow peas, chopped

1 large carro,t chopped

1 cup broccoli, chopped

1 cup bean sprouts

1½ teaspoons fresh grated ginger root

1 clove garlic chopped

1 tablespoon soy sauce

1 tablespoon olive oil

Method:

Cut the chicken into small pieces. Heat the oil in a wok until very hot add all the ingredients and stir continuously until chicken is cooked and vegetables should still be firm and crunchy.

Oven Temperatures

	Celsius	Fahrenheit	Gas Mark
Very Slow	120	250	1
Slow	150	300	2
Moderately slow	160	325	3
Moderate	180 – 190	350 – 375	4
Moderately hot	200 – 210	400 – 425	5
Hot	220 – 230	450 – 475	6
Very hot	240 - 250	500 - 525	7

EDIBLE FLOWERS

Flowers can make a colourful finishing touch to any salad and there are many that are perfectly safe to eat. Make sure you wash them carefully to remove any little birds calling cards, insects and the possibility of a bee hiding amongst the petals. If you intend to use flowers for decorating salads don't use any pesticide or fungicide and make sure sprays from your neighbors garden have not drifted onto them.

Flowers that are safe to eat:

Calendula: The orange or yellow petals can be sprinkled over a salad they have a peppery taste.

Chrysanthemum: The petals are similar to calendula and can be used in the same way.

Day Lily: They only last for one day hence the name. They come in yellow, pink, cream, mauve and bronze. Pinch out their green sepals and use them whole or shredded.

Elderflower: They have small white flowers on a large head in spring. The flowers can be used to flavour champagne; the berries are used to make wine and jellies.

Fruit blossoms: The petals of cherries, plums, peaches, apples, crab apples and all the citrus make lightly flavoured garnishes for salads.

Geranium & Pelargonium: Can be used as decoration on salads. The scented leaves release flavour when added during cooking.

Herb flowers: Basil, parsley, mint, marjoram and chives can be added as garnishes.

Honeysuckle: Remove the calyx and shred the petals, they have a lightly honeyed flavour and perfume.

Lavender: There are many varieties and all can be used, milled into sugar and mixed into ice cream, biscuits and jams.

Marigolds: Can be used in the same way as calendula.

Nasturtiums: The flower, leaves and seeds can be used to garnish a salad. They have a slightly peppery taste; the seeds are very hot the flowers and leaves are quite mild.

Rose: They make a wonderful garnish for any salad, be careful to wash them thoroughly to get rid of any pesticides or bees.

Vegetable flowers: The blossoms of peas, beans, lettuce and male zucchini and pumpkin make a nice garnish for salads. The bitter stamen should be pinched out before eating.

Violet, Viola and Pansy: The bright colours make an excellent garnish for salads.

PULSES & GRAINS

Beans, peas and lentils (collectively known as pulses) need soaking before use. They should be placed into a container and covered with water for 8 hours; if they are soaked for longer they may ferment. After draining and washing they can be boiled in water or frozen for future use.

Barley, pearl: The outer husk (bran) has been removed and the grain has been steamed and polished. There is no need to soak pearl barley it cooks in 30 minutes.

Black-eyed beans: Small kidney-shaped beans , cream coloured, with little black markings like eyes. Soak them overnight and cook for 30 minutes.

Borlotti beans: Large kidney-shaped beans, beige to brown with dark red speckles that disappear when cooked. Soak overnight and cook for 1 ½ hours.

Kidney beans: Dark red kidney-shaped beans. Soak overnight boil for 10 minutes then simmer for 30 minutes.

Pinto beans: These are like small borlotti beans. Soak overnight and cook for 1 ¼ hours.

Burghul: Also called cracked wheat and bulghur. To cook pour boiling water over it and stand for 15 minutes then drain well.

Chickpeas: Also called garbanzo or ceci beans. Soak overnight and cook for 1 hour.

Lentils: Red lentils do not require soaking, cook for 10 minutes. Soak brown lentils (also called green) overnight and cook for 45 minutes.

Polenta: Also known as cornmeal, boil in water or milk for 20 minutes. Eat it as it is or spread it out to dry then cut it into shapes and fry it.

Arborio rice: Large round-grained rice that absorbs liquid well without turning too soft. Suitable for risottos, it takes about 35 minutes to cook.

Basmati rice: A thin white fragrant long- grained rice; wash before cooking. Cooks in 15 minutes.

Brown rice: A short-grained rice cooks in 30 minutes.

White rice: Available in long or short grains, cooks in 15 minutes.

Wild rice: It is really a seed from an aquatic grass; it has a nutty flavour and chewy texture. Cook for 30 minutes.

Split peas: There is no need to soak them, yellow split peas take 30 minutes to cook. Green split peas take about 1 ½ hours to cook.

Rice varieties:

Arborio (low GI)	Wild rice
Jasmine	Basmati (low GI)
White glutinous	Brown long-grain
White short-grain	Black glutinous
Brown short-grain	Brown rice & wild rice blend

Leafy Greens:

Lettuce;

Rocket	Radicchio
Green coral	Mesclun
Red mignonette	Red coral
Curly endive	Iceberg
Butter lettuce	Mizuna

Cos lettuce	Baby cos lettuce
Red oak leaf	Lamb's lettuce
Green oak leaf	Red & white Belgian endive

Vegetable greens;

Baby spinach	Spinach
Silverbeet (Swiss chard)	Cabbage
Brussels sprouts	

Asian greens;

Bok Choy	Baby bok choy
Kangkung	Choy sum
Gai larn	Tat soi

Sprouted seeds:

Mustard	Watercress
Mung beans	Snow pea
Alfalfa	

Herbs;

Coriander	Basil
Flat parsley	Curly parsley
Mint	Chocolate mint
Oregano	Rosemary
Sage	Tarragon
Bay leaves	Thyme
Dill	Lemon grass
Marjoram	Chervil

Mushrooms;

Shitake	Flat
Button	Cremini
Chinese	

Rice products;

Flat rice noodles	Rice noodle sheets

Rice vermicelli

Rice paper

Rice flakes

Rice cakes

Nuts;

Flaked almonds

Slivered almonds

Blanched almonds

Ground almonds

Hazelnuts

Pecans

Pistachios

Macadamias

Pine nuts

Peanuts

Cashews

Walnuts

Brazil nuts

Home Made Stock

Vegetable Stock;

4 bay leaves

2 large carrots, chopped

2 large parsnips, chopped

4 medium onions, chopped

12 sticks of celery

2 teaspoons black peppercorns

6 litres water (24 cups)

Vegetable Stock; Method;

Combine all ingredients in a large pan, simmer uncovered for 1 ½ hours; strain. The stock can be frozen in batches and stored for up to 6 months, Makes about 2.5 litres (10 cups).

Beef stock:

2 kg meaty beef bones

2 medium onions, chopped

2 sticks of celery, chopped

2 medium carrots, chopped

3 bay leaves

2 teaspoons black peppercorns

5 litres (20cups) water

3 litres (12 cups) extra water

Beef stock: Method;

Fish stock:

1.5 kg fish bones

3 litres (12 cups) water

1 medium onion, chopped

2 sticks celery, chopped

2 bay leaves

1 teaspoon of black peppercorns

Fish stock: Method;

Combine all the ingredients in a large pan and simmer uncovered for 20 minutes, strain.

Combine all ingredients into a large pan and simmer uncovered for 4 hrs add extra water and simmer for another hour uncovered, strain. Can be frozen.

All stock recipes make about 2.5 litres of stock.

Chicken stock:

2 kg chicken bones

2 medium onions, chopped

2 sticks of celery, chopped

2 medium carrots, chopped

3 bay leaves

2 teaspoons black peppercorns

5 litres (20 cups) water

Chicken stock: Method;

Combine all ingredients in large pan and simmer for 2 hrs, strain.

Home Made Salad Dressings

No fat salad dressings:

Soy & ginger;

¼ cup of rice vinegar

2 tablespoons light soy sauce

1 tablespoon lemon juice

2 teaspoons brown sugar

½ teaspoon grated fresh ginger

Makes ½ a cup.

Sweet chilli dressing;

¼ cup of rice vinegar

2 tablespoons sweet chilli sauce

1 teaspoon fish sauce

1 teaspoon finely chopped fresh coriander

Makes ½ a cup.

Mustard & honey dressing;

1 tablespoon of honey

¼ cup of orange juice

2 teaspoons seeded mustard

1 teaspoon finely chopped thyme

Salad dressings:

French dressing;

Half a cup of white vinegar

¾ cup of olive oil

½ teaspoon of brown sugar

1 teaspoon of Dijon mustard

Makes 1 cup

Fresh tomato sauce;

3 large tomatoes, peeled, seeded & chopped

2 green onions chopped

1/3 cup of red wine vinegar

1/3 cup of sweet chilli sauce

2 cloves of garlic chopped

1 teaspoon seeded mustard

1 teaspoon brown sugar

Fresh tomato sauce continued

1 teaspoon cracked black pepper

¼ cup of chopped fresh parsley

Makes 1 ¼ cups

Italian dressing;

Makes ½ a cup.

Garlic balsamic dressing;

1 medium bulb of garlic

1 tablespoon of balsamic vinegar

¼ cup of white wine vinegar

2 teaspoons of brown sugar

Makes ½ a cup.

Guilt-free dressing

½ cup of buttermilk

2 tablespoon finely chopped fresh chives

2 tablespoons of no-oil French dressing

1 tablespoon seeded mustard

1 tablespoon of honey

Makes 2/3 cup

2 tablespoons white wine vinegar

2 tablespoons lemon juice

½ teaspoon of brown sugar

2 cloves of garlic crushed

¾ cup of olive oil

1 tablespoon finely chopped fresh basil

1 tablespoon finely chopped fresh oregano.

Makes 1 cup

Method:

For each dressing combine ingredients in a container with a lid and shake well, or use a blender.

Mayonnaise;

Basic mayonnaise;

2 egg yolks

1 tablespoon of lemon juice

½ teaspoon of salt

½ teaspoon of dry mustard

¾ cup of light olive oil

Method:

Blend egg yolks, juice, salt & mustard until smooth. Add oil and blend until the sauce is thick. Makes ¾ cup.

Thousand island mayonnaise;

1/3 cup of tomato paste

1/3 cup of tomato sauce

1 tablespoon of Worcestershire sauce

½ teaspoon of Tabasco sauce

¾ cup of basic mayonnaise.

Method:

Blend the ingredients together. Makes 1 ¼ cups.

Curried mayonnaise;

1 tablespoon of curry powder

¾ cup of basic mayonnaise

Add powder to a dry pan stir until fragrant .

Method:

Blend into basic mayonnaise. Makes ¾ cup

Herb mayonnaise;

2 tablespoons chopped fresh chives

2 tablespoons chopped fresh parsley

2 tablespoons chopped fresh basil leaves

¾ cup of basic mayonnaise

Method:

Blend herbs into basic mayonnaise. Makes ¾ cup.

Garlic mayonnaise;

3 cloves of garlic chopped

¾ cup of basic mayonnaise

Method:

Blend garlic with basic mayonnaise. Makes ¾ cup.

Tomato Sauce:

1/3 cup of olive oil

4 small onions finely, chopped

20 medium tomatoes

8 cloves of garlic, crushed

2/3 cup of chopped fresh basil leaves

salt & pepper to taste

Tomato Sauce: Method;

Heat the oil in a large pan, add onions, cover and cook over a low heat for 20 minutes, stirring occasionally.

Meanwhile peel seed and chop the tomatoes, discard stem ends.

Add the garlic to the pan and cook for 5 minutes. Add the tomatoes and bring to the boil reduce heat and simmer for 1 ½ hours stir in basil and continue cooking for another 10 minutes. Add seasoning to taste, cool and pour into freezer containers keeps for up to 6 months. Makes 2.5 litres.

Semi-dried Tomatoes;

Place tomatoes cut in half on an oven rack in an oven dish in a very slow oven for about 2 hrs. Store for up to 5 days in a covered container with a little olive oil in the refrigerator.

Drying Tomatoes:

There are two methods of drying tomatoes; oven dried and sun dried. The best tomatoes to use are Roma or egg tomatoes. If using larger tomatoes cut them into quarters.

Good sunny days with little air moisture is needed for sun drying. If these conditions cannot be guaranteed oven drying is better. **Sun drying;** Place tomatoes cut in half on a rack in a deep baking dish in the sunniest position possible. Dry fresh thyme or oregano for extra flavour when bottling. Drying takes 3 to 4 days, bring tomatoes indoors at night.

Oven drying; Place tomatoes cut in half on racks in baking dishes and place in a very slow oven for up to 8 hours, thyme and oregano may be dried at the same time for

Oven drying;

the first 30 minutes to add flavour when the tomatoes are bottled.

Pack into sterilized jars cover with olive oil and add herbs. Keep in a cool dark place, once opened keep in the refrigerator. The oil can be used for cooking if kept in the refrigerator for up to 1 week.

How To Cook Rice

Absorption (Steamed) Method;

Combine water and rice in a medium heavy-based pan, cover tightly, bring to the boil, reduce heat to as low as possible, cook for recommended time. Do not remove lid during cooking time. Remove pan from the heat, let it stand covered for 10 minutes.

Microwave Method;

Combine rice and boiling water in a large microwave-safe bowl or jug. Cook uncovered on HIGH for recommended time or until rice is tender. Stir halfway through cooking. Cover and let it stand for 5 minutes.

Baked Method;

Combine rice and boiling water in an ovenproof dish, stir well. Cover tightly with foil or a lid. Bake in a moderate oven for recommended time or until rice is tender.

Boiled Method;

Bring the water to the boil in a large pan, add rice, stir to separate the grains, boil uncovered for recommended time or until the rice is tender.

Do not rinse cooked rice unless it is specified in the recipe.

Electric rice cookers or rice steamers give good consistent results.

Rice tips;

One cup of uncooked brown or white rice =200g

One cup of uncooked wild rice = 180g

White rice almost triples in bulk during cooking, brown and wild rice double in bulk.

Store uncooked rice in a tightly covered container in a cool dark place.

Left over cooked rice will keep covered in the refrigerator for 2 days or in the freezer for 2 months.

Bibliography

Bullivant V. DSc: DNM. 'The Natural Way To Better Health and Longer Life.

Cabot S. MD. 'Don't Let Your Hormones Ruin Your Life' Women's Health Advisory Service.

Coli T. Miller M. et al Editors. 'Fruit 'n' Veg With Every Meal' JB Fairfax Pty Ltd.

Clements A. BA: MD: BCh: DPH(Syd): MPHc (Calif). Et al. Editor. 'Infant And Family Health In Australia' Longman Group Ltd.

Diamond H & M. 'Fit For Life' Angus And Robertson.

Earl R. PhD, Imrie D. MD. Et al. 'Your Vitality Quotient' Warner Books.

Fergusson C. FRCS: COS: et al. 'Your Active Body' Harrap Books.

Horne R. Bobbin T. 'The Health Revolution' Golden Press Pty Ltd.

Hunter J. MD. et al. 'The Allergy Diet' Methuen Australia Pty Ltd.

Martini F.PhD. 'Fundamentals Of Anatomy And Physiology' Prentice Hall Inc.

Papalia D.E. PhD: et al. 'Life Span Development' Mc Graw-Hill Book Company Australia Pty Ltd.

Samra G. MB: BS: MD. 'The Hypoglycemic Connection' M.I.N.T. Enterprises.

Toon P. GP. et al. 'Your heart And Lungs' Harrap Books Ltd.

Ward B. et al. 'Your Diet' Harrap Publishing Group.

Wentworth J.A. 'The Migraine Guide And Cook Book' Sidgwick & Jackson Ltd.

Brand Miller Dr J. et al. 'The GI Factor, The Glucose Revolution' Hodder Headline 2nd Edition.

Anne Rogers has also written

Renewal (Supernatural/ Fantasy) short story

The Fatal Planet (Science Fiction) short story

The Shift Worker (poetry)

Mission 14 (Science Fiction) Novel

River Crossing (Science Fiction) Novel

Prince And The Apple Tree (childrens picture book)

Captain Dan And Sailor Sam (childrens picture book)

Sooty Wooty Is A Cat (childrens picture book)

The Legend of the Sun Kitten (childrens picture book)

Anne Rogers would like to thank

Peter and Jenny Herriman for

Web page and computer support

Editors:

Jayne Stokes

Anastasia Cassella-Young

About the author

Anne Rogers

Anne Rogers is a South Australian fiction author, a poet and children's picture book author and illustrator. Over the years she has written many stories and will continue to write many more. Anne completed and published a book on healthy eating last year. Visit Anne's website http://annerogers.websouth.com.au Anne has been a 'Jack of all Trades' during her lifetime, working in the spinning and weaving industries making Axminster carpets, bookbinding, electrical fittings, plastic moldings and plant irrigation. She has diploma's in esthetics, nutrition and massage and worked in the Health Care profession. Anne has a lifelong love of horses and cats. In England she competed in horse trials at international level, show jumping and dressage with the horses she bred and trained, only giving up due to a fall from one of her horses, when she injured her back seriously. She bred pedigree cats after coming to Australia only giving that up in order to devote all her time to writing and illustrating her books. Anne was born in Gloucestershire England in 1946. At the age of 5 her parents immigrated to Sydney Australia. When she was 11 the family moved back to Gloucestershire. In 1983 Anne returned to Australia to live in Adelaide, South Australia. Later in 1997 she moved from the city to the peace of the country side.
Anne is a retired nurse and qualified nutritionist. She spent 10 years researching this book. She was very overweight, 18 stone while nursing and was desperate to lose weight. Anne tried lots of diets, which failed. She decided to research and write this book after qualifying as a nutritionist; she lost weight by putting the advice in the book in to practice. Anne now weighs 10.5 stone and feels better. She does not diet and eats as much as she wants and enjoys her food and her new found health. Many people have benefited from the book and have improved their health.

Anne Rogers Author of Children's Books, Fiction for all Ages, Poetry, and Children's Book Illustrator. Australian buyers can purchase Anne's Book's, Calendar's, CD's, and greeting cards directly from her in Australia, save money and pay Australian postage rates. Go to her personal website, for all the details. Website: www.annerogers.net

Disclaimer: The author of this book does not in anyway guarantee that a person will lose weight, improve their energy levels or health. Everyone has a different metabolic rate and this may effect their individual success in achieving their goal. Results will also depend on how well they follow the guide lines in this book. Also people with a medical condition effecting their health weight or energy levels may experience different results from those obtained by other people. Certain prescription drugs can effect weight loss and it may be necessary to cut down on the amount of food consumed and/or take more exercise to gain satisfactory results.